Configuring Contagion

Series: Epistemologies of Healing
General Editors: David Parkin and Elisabeth Hsu: both are at ISCA, Oxford

This series publishes monographs and edited volumes on indigenous (so-called traditional) medical knowledge and practice, alternative and complementary medicine, and ethnobiological studies that relate to health and illness. The emphasis of the series is on the way indigenous epistemologies inform healing, against a background of comparison with other practices, and in recognition of the fluidity between them.

Recent volumes:

Volume 19
Configuring Contagion: Ethnographies of Biosocial Epidemics
Edited by Lotte Meinert and Jens Seeberg

Volume 18
Fierce Medicines, Fragile Socialities: Grounding Global HIV Treatment in Tanzania
Dominik Mattes

Volume 17
Capturing Quicksilver: The Position, Power, and Plasticity of Chinese Medicine in Singapore
Arielle A. Smith

Volume 16
Ritual Retellings: Luangan Healing Performances through Practice
Isabell Herrmans

Volume 15
Healing Roots: Anthropology in Life and Medicine
Julie Laplante

Volume 14
Asymmetrical Conversations: Contestations, Circumventions, and the Blurring of Therapeutic Boundaries
Edited by Harish Naraindas, Johannes Quack, and William S. Sax

Volume 13
The Body in Balance: Humoral Medicines in Practice
Edited by Peregrine Horden and Elisabeth Hsu

Volume 12
Manufacturing Tibetan Medicine: The Creation of an Industry and the Moral Economy of Tibetanness
Martin Saxer

Volume 11
Fortune and the Cursed: The Sliding Scale of Time in Mongolian Divination
Katherine Swancutt

Volume 10
Medicine between Science and Religion: Explorations on Tibetan Grounds
Edited by Vincanne Adams, Mona Schrempf, and Sienna R. Craig

For a full volume listing, please see the series page on our website:
https://www.berghahnbooks.com/series/epistemologies-of-healing

Configuring Contagion
Ethnographies of Biosocial Epidemics

Edited by Lotte Meinert and Jens Seeberg

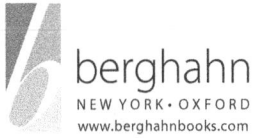

berghahn
NEW YORK·OXFORD
www.berghahnbooks.com

First published in 2022 by
Berghahn Books
www.berghahnbooks.com

© 2022, 2025 Lotte Meinert and Jens Seeberg
First paperback edition published in 2025

All rights reserved. Except for the quotation of short passages
for the purposes of criticism and review, no part of this book
may be reproduced in any form or by any means, electronic or
mechanical, including photocopying, recording, or any information
storage and retrieval system now known or to be invented,
without written permission of the publisher.

Library of Congress Cataloging-in-Publication Data

Names: Meinert, Lotte, editor. | Seeberg, Jens, editor.
Title: Configuring contagion : ethnographies of biosocial epidemics / edited by Lotte Meinert and Jens Seeberg.
Description: First edition. | New York : Berghahn Books, 2022. | Series: Epistemologies of healing ; 19 | Includes bibliographical references and index.
Identifiers: LCCN 2021028790 (print) | LCCN 2021028791 (ebook) | ISBN 9781800733046 (hardback) | ISBN 9781800733053 (ebook)
Subjects: LCSH: Epidemics--Philosophy. | Epidemics--Research. | Epidemics--Social aspects. | Epidemics--Political aspects. | COVID-19 (Disease)
Classification: LCC RA648.5 .C66 2022 (print) | LCC RA648.5 (ebook) | DDC 614.4--dc23
LC record available at https://lccn.loc.gov/2021028790
LC ebook record available at https://lccn.loc.gov/2021028791

British Library Cataloguing in Publication Data
A catalogue record for this book is available from the British Library

ISBN 978-1-80073-304-6 hardback
ISBN 978-1-80539-727-4 paperback
ISBN 978-1-80539-914-8 epub
ISBN 978-1-80073-305-3 web pdf

https://doi.org/10.3167/9781800733046

Contents

List of Figures	vii
Introduction. Configuring Contagion in Biosocial Epidemics Lotte Meinert and Jens Seeberg	1
1. Gender Configurations and Suicide in Northern Uganda Susan Reynolds Whyte and Henry Oboke	23
2. Configuring Epidemic Suicide in Oceania Edward Lowe	44
3. Haunted by the Future: Autism and the Spectre of Prison – Configuring Race and Disability in the African American Community Cheryl Mattingly and Stephanie Keeney Parks	68
4. Configuring Affection: Family Experiences of Obesity and Social Contagion in Denmark Lone Grøn	100
5. Health Activists and Trauma Contagion: Cultural Epidemics and Raising Awareness of Trauma in Post-conflict, Post-tsunami Aceh Jesse Hession Grayman, Mary-Jo DelVecchio Good and Byron J. Good	124
6. Touched by Violence: Configuring Affliction after War in Northern Uganda Lars Williams and Lotte Meinert	144
7. 'These Spirit Attacks Are Like an Epidemic': Spirit Possession as Affective Contagion in Niger Adeline Masquelier, Abouzeidi Maidouka Dillé and Ly Amadou H. Belko	166

8. Haunted by Internet Porn: Configuration of a Hidden
   Contagion   193
   Douglas Hollan

9. Contagious Configurations: Reproductive Governance
   from Abortion to Zika Virus in Latin America   213
   Lynn M. Morgan

10. Figures of Drug-Resistant Tuberculosis   228
    *Jens Seeberg, Bijayalaxmi Rautaray and
    Shyama Mohapatra*

Afterword. Epidemics and Ghosts   248
   Byron J. Good

Index   259

Figures

4.1. 'Conviction 6' by Maria Speyer.
Photo by and courtesy of Maria Speyer,
www.mariaspeyer.com.   101

4.2. Rita's drawing of her family and friend network.
Persons marked with stars are considered obese
by Rita. Photo by Tove Nyholm.   106

4.3. Karsten and Tina's drawing of their family and
friend network. Persons underlined are considered
obese by Karsten and Tina. Photo by Tove Nyholm.   109

4.4. Susanne's drawing of her family and friend network.
Persons marked with circles (red in the original
drawing) are considered obese by Susanne.
Photo by Tove Nyholm.   112

4.5. Peter, Mette, Hannah, Sussie and Stefanie's drawing
of their family and friend network. Persons marked
with circles (red in the original drawing) are
considered obese by them. Photo by Tove Nyholm.   116

Introduction
Configuring Contagion in Biosocial Epidemics

Lotte Meinert and Jens Seeberg

How do epidemics spread? The short, standard answer is through contagion. For most infectious disease epidemics, we are well aware that this happens through the transfer of microbes between people or between animals and humans. The COVID-19 pandemic has made this clear all around the globe, and many people have become increasingly aware of epidemic dynamics and concepts. Yet not all epidemics can be attributed to infection. A large part of the global burden of disease is due to so-called noncommunicable diseases.[1] How do these and other non-infectious conditions spread? Can they even be termed epidemic and contagious? This book offers ways to think about and expand our understanding of contagion beyond typical notions of infectious pandemics, beyond viral emergencies, to include the larger field of biosocial epidemics. Fundamentally we challenge the notion of noncommunicability (Seeberg and Meinert 2015), as it seems to render the epidemic spread of other forms of disease impossible. Some researchers have even proposed that we stop using the category of noncommunicable disease (Adjaye-Gbewonyo and Vaughan 2019; Blundell and Hine 2018) because many of these diseases are in fact communicable. In this book, we propose varied and detailed answers to questions about the epidemic and contagious potentials of specific infections and non-infectious conditions. We explore how inseparable social and biological processes configure co-existing influences which create epidemics, and we stress the role of social inequality in these processes. We use the term biosocial – in one word and without a hyphen – to underline that these processes are indivisible. Epidemics do not spread evenly in populations and simply through coincidental biological contagion. They are socially structured and selective, and contagion happens under specific economic, political and environmental conditions in which various influences configure to make contagion possible. Even though this book is mainly – but not entirely – about so-called non-infectious diseases, we dwell for a moment on the corona pandemic because it underlines that something we usually perceive as entirely biological is in fact biosocial. Likewise, what we may assume to be fully social has inseparable biological sides.

The rapid escalation of the Severe Acute Respiratory Syndrome Coronavirus 2 (SARS-CoV-2), also known as new coronavirus, from its initial outbreak in Wuhan, China, into pandemic proportions in early 2020, is a good example of biosocial contagion. A virus does not constitute a form of life in itself but may be said to exist at the border of life. Coronavirus is an RNA virus and so depends on access to a living cell in which it can copy itself. It does not qualify as a species but may be considered as a quasi-species (Eigen, McCaskill and Schuster 1989) and, like influenza, it may jump between species and affect them in the process to become what Celia Low has termed a 'species multiplier' (Lowe 2010). In biosocial terms, it is a string of information whose existence depends on communication – a basic form of exchange that constitutes sociality – between human and/or non-human becomings (Ingold 2013). Indeed, the zoonotic origin of the human experience of hosting the virus is linked to the intensified social interaction between human and non-human species that were previously in less frequent contact in densely populated urban spaces, as exemplified by the original epicentre of the coronavirus epidemic, the now famous Huanan Seafood Wholesale Market in Wuhan, China. In other words, coronavirus cannot be understood as purely biological because it could not exist outside the realm of the social. Coronavirus is intrinsically biosocial. Whereas the theoretical implications of this fact have been somewhat overlooked during the pandemic, its ramifications for global control measures are obvious. All over the globe, barriers have been created to block the biosocial interaction between virus and humans through the political regulation of human social life by way of physical distancing, quarantine, improved hygiene and the adoption of facial masks as well as through wider societal lockdowns of workplaces, sectors such as education, cities, regions and countries, disallowing most forms of physical movement and engagement. The combined impact of new coronavirus and strict control measures has reconfigured pre-existing vulnerabilities. In India, a strict societal lockdown with only four hours' warning sent millions of migrant workers on the move away from urban centres to rural places of origin, risking a rapid nationwide spread of the virus (Maji, Choudhari and Sushma 2020) and leaving desperate migrants without access to food or healthcare. People with chronic conditions such as diabetes in need of treatment experienced interrupted access to care due to either self-isolation or fear of COVID-19, or because healthcare services did not function as usual. Such dynamics had the potential to turn (the risk of) co-morbidities into new syndemics (see below), as coronavirus and its control came to interact with other epidemics along socioeconomic faultlines. We have not yet seen the full impact of the variations of configuring coronavirus-cum-control measures across and within countries, but it is likely that other public health concerns such as tuberculosis (TB) control have been severely affected, with a risk of widespread treatment interruption potentially leading to a surge in multidrug-resistant TB. Whereas the present volume does not address the coronavirus pandemic as such, since the book had been nearly completed prior to this event, we believe that it provides important contributions that may inspire future explorations of this pandemic and future ones.

Epidemics

Our conception of epidemics is a specific one. There are at least two senses of the term epidemic: (1) The standard epidemiological definition of an epidemic as the rapid spread of infectious disease to an unusually large number of people in a given population within a short period of time (see, e.g., Center for Disease Control[2]); (2) The wider use of the term in public discourse as a metaphor for something – often alarming – that seems to have arisen quickly. The term 'epidemic' has been applied to the spread of noncommunicable diseases, such as cancer and obesity (Martin and Martin-Granel 2006: 979) in a metaphorical sense (Moffat 2010), thereby assuming a distinction between 'real' epidemics involving the spread of infection, and *quasi* epidemics which are postmodern and socially constructed (Boero 2007; Grøn and Meinert 2017). Our use of the term epidemic refers to the spread of infectious and non-infectious diseases alike, and our use of the term is not simply metaphorical; we are interested in phenomena – of many different kinds – that actually spread in epidemic patterns, and in how this happens. In other words, we are interested in the factual and practical levels of how various communicable and non-communicable diseases spread epidemically. Rather than limiting the term epidemic to infectious diseases and using the term in a strictly metaphorical sense about other phenomena, we explore what we claim are actual epidemic patterns. With the concept of biosocial contagion, various vernacular terms for and understandings of spread and social influence, as well as theoretical conceptions such as imitation (Tarde 1903), affect (Stewart 2007) and resonance (Rosa 2019), we seek to widen the terminology employed to talk about the biosocial configuration of epidemics. This conception of epidemics enables us to explore how phenomena such as obesity, spirit possession, ADHD, suicide, trauma and some forms of cancer spread in certain populations at particular times, and to develop new insights into how these processes transpire.

Epidemics of various kinds always involve some kind of contagion, and are often configured by more than one kind of contagion and social influence that result in disease. For analytical purposes, we can distinguish roughly between biological kinds of contagion and social kinds of contagion. In reality, however, biological and social contagion are fundamentally inseparable. It is well known that infectious disease epidemics such as HIV and TB interweave biological factors such as viral, bacterial and fungal influences with factors such as human nutrition, gender relations, health system dynamics and phenomena such as love. Epidemics of non-infectious diseases like ADHD, autism and PTSD may not involve biological contagion as such, but they are biosocial phenomena that simultaneously involve forms of social and biological influence that in turn have biological and social consequences.

Diagnostic systems may in themselves contribute to the creation of what could be called 'epidemics of attention' regarding diseases such as ADHD or cancer. However, diagnostic attention can seldom account for an entire epidemic. There are usually other dynamics at work as well. Some of the dynamics involved in epidemic phenomena such as suicide, self-harm, spirit possession, alcoholism and depression may involve social contagion processes such as affect, inspiration, aspiration and haunting (Folmann 2017; Nielsen 2017). Social, historical and political circumstances are always part of the configuration of a contagious landscape that influences members of social groups in various ways. An example of this is lung cancer, which is an epidemic in areas where the industrial production and promotion of tobacco is widespread, political regulation has been minimal, and smoking is regarded by particular population groups as socially attractive, and may later turn into addiction for some. Another example of how (the lack of) political regulation plays a significant role in the prevention or development of epidemics is the obesity epidemic and the way in which the industrial production and commercialization of food and beverages at particular places and points in history clearly influence the spread of obesity (see Grøn, this volume). Short-term as well as long-term political awareness and regulation or ignorance and laissez-faire policy clearly influence environmental factors, including those that lead to climate change – which affects health conditions as well. For some time now, we have been aware of how climate change influences the distribution of mosquitos and the risk of vector-borne diseases such as malaria, dengue fever and Zika virus (see Morgan, this volume). There is now also growing awareness of how climate change influences the spread of conditions such as asthma, anaemia, heart disease and depression (Coleman and Littlejohn 2019). The occurrence of (new) epidemics, including those that cross the problematic boundary between communicable epidemics and noncommunicable epidemics, calls into question what drives or slows down such epidemics and what configurations of contagion are at work in these processes.

Epidemics are the biosocial consequences of unique configurations of circumstances incorporating phenomena that are both biological and social. They are products of interconnections and interactions – they are epigenetic, intersubjective and contextual processes that happen over time. In this book we reflect on epidemic phenomena through the concepts of biosocial contagion and configuration to emphasize systemic relations between different kinds of contagious and contaminating processes. The chapters in this book challenge and rethink the concepts of contagion and configuration in relation to specific diseases, conditions and social phenomena.

We build upon the medical historian Charles Rosenberg's distinction between configuration and contamination explanations (Rosenberg 1992). As a historian, Rosenberg described two kinds of explanatory models in time: (1) Configuration views that conceptualized epidemics as disturbing climatic and social balances which maintained health; and (2) contamination views that tended towards biological reductionism and placed emphasis on person-to-person contagion and micro-organisms. This notion of contagion was gradually eliminated from biomedical discourse as a result of the discovery of microbiological infectants, such as bacteria, which led to the creation of the category of 'infectious diseases' (Pernick 2002). In this book, we work towards an anti-reductionistic return to the concept of contagion seen as a biosocial recovery of the idea of infection as embedded in its wider societal configuration. We propose analytical combinations of contagion and configuration theories, and we consider how local and regional epistemologies conceptualize the spread and causation of disease and epidemics. We apply Singer and Clair's (2003) important concept of syndemic, which indicates how various epidemics often play out together and are closely integrated – such as HIV, TB and certain forms of cancer, which are often defined as merely co-morbidity (Livingston 2020), or PTSD and depression, which often seem to accompany each other. This syndemic approach to health challenges conventional historical understandings of diseases as distinct entities in nature, separate from other diseases and independent of social contexts and environmental factors (Singer et al. 2017). The chapters in this book explore specific syndemic processes through a combination of experience-near approaches to the configuring of contagion in everyday lives, and analysis of how socioeconomic structures and social inequality shape syndemics. The chapters also explore how specific local epistemologies conceptualize and contribute to the configuring of such processes. We describe the two central concepts of contagion and configuration in some detail below, followed by a brief description of the chapters in the book.

Contagion

The discovery of micro-organisms as pathogens meant that the term 'contagious disease' became too broad and imprecise, and medical science opted for the more specific term 'infectious disease'. We suggest that we reconsider the term 'contagious' – not only when it is applied to disease, but also with regard to other phenomena (Fainzang 1996; Matthews 1968). We invoke and apply a broad and inclusive understanding of biosocial contagious processes because various epidemic phenomena and circumstances often happen in syndemic processes (Singer and Clair 2003) in which multiple epidemic phenomena, local epistemologies and socioeconomic, political and ecological circumstances work together.

Social contagion may describe various kinds of processes in which entities influence each other 'with touch' (from the Latin *con tangere*). These entities may be minds and mindful bodies (Scheper-Hughes and Lock 1987), body parts or larger entities of families, friends, communities or organizations. Gabriel Tarde's early study of imitation from 1903 is notable in relation to social contagion because his most basic and radical idea was that sociality is imitation, and he describes some of these processes of social influence as contagion.[3] Tarde wrote about the triad of imitation (repetition), opposition (to imitation) and invention. He regarded imitation as the most common social form. He rejected ideas about oppositions such as subject-object and individual-society, and he regarded imitation as neither voluntary nor involuntary, but as a basic and universal dynamic of society. One of Tarde's main contributions to our understanding of contagion is his point about how imitation happens between two or more units of analysis. Imitation is not necessarily intentional or directed, and the process is as much about the responding part (the imitator) as the imitated. Tarde's interest in what might be termed the elementary structures of (social) processes is potentially useful for thinking about how contagion happens. Tarde pointed to the way in which currents of imitation happen over time – in history as well as in molecular processes of vibration. He saw all social resemblance as repetition, and wrote: 'repetitions are also multiplications or self-spreading contagions. If a stone falls into the water, the first wave which it produces will repeat itself in circling out to the confines of its basin'

(Tarde 1903: 17). In his view, imitation is what drives diffusion and infusion, but it does so in diverse environments and is influenced by other waves. Waves affect each other and create interferences. We find Tarde's early ideas useful for thinking about how various forms of biosocial contagion and influence happen in practice and can be configured into biosocial epidemics. If we think about contagion as a form of communication, Gregory Bateson's famous insight that 'we cannot not communicate' becomes relevant. The idea that some diseases are 'noncommunicable' seems unlikely, because disease will always influence the system of which it is part (Bateson [1972] 2000). Bateson's systemic thinking in relation to selves, families, ecologies and minds and how they influence each other speaks directly to the perspective we cultivate in this book.

Social contagion processes often involve influence in the form of affect (Grøn 2017), responses to phenomena to which we cannot not respond (Waldenfels 2011), resonance (Rosa 2019), moods (Throop 2017), violence (Meinert and Whyte 2017), haunting (Good 2015; Meinert 2019), stigma (Lawlor and Solomon 2017; Mattingly 2017), and processes of imitation and diversification (Hollan 2017). The entities which influence each other may sometimes be hard to delineate: where does one self begin and another stop? Where is the limit between an individual and a group? Some forms of social contagion tend to run in the family through kinship connections (Meinert and Grøn 2019). Kinship connections highlight the fact that contagion is often ambivalent and tricky to deal with because it involves both positive and negative influence and nutritious and poisonous aspects (ibid.). Contagious kinship connections happen through various processes of belonging (Grøn 2019), child witnessing (Han and Brandel 2019), fear (Seeberg 2019; Stevenson 2019), love (Garcia 2014, 2019), and bitterness and affection (Oboke and Whyte 2019). Attempts to deal with contagious kinship connections may involve family therapy (Kuan 2019) or making cuts in physical bodies and family relations (Grøn 2019). Processes of social contagion may be unspecific and diffuse like the subconscious impact of subtle advertisements, yet when contagious processes happen there is often no doubt that they take place – we find ourselves buying products we have seen in advertisements, as do our friends – and we experience their effects, sometimes in the form of large-scale epidemics.

Introduction

Whereas contagion often concerns processes involving human and non-human actors, sometimes connected in zoonotic epidemics, the concept of contamination involves a process (of a substance) that spreads in an environment, often with some kind of pollution being involved, at a pace which may be either rapid or diffuse and slow. Contaminating and contaminated areas may be large-scale, such as the environment, the market, the food industry or the pharmaceutical industry, but at the same time processes of contamination may be subtle, involving slow, poisonous contact, or marketing strategies directed towards permeable selves or bodies. Social contamination may involve processes of environmental influence, such as when the atmosphere in a room or the history in a landscape touches or affects us (Grøn and Meinert 2017). Processes of social contagion and contamination are contingent upon the perceived permeability of selves (Napier 2013; Taylor 1989; Throop 2017) and mindful bodies (Scheper-Hughes and Lock 1987); and upon the way in which social, historical and environmental influences saturate subjectivities and materialities. Actors – individuals, families, institutions, states – may take action to attempt to create protection against contamination, and may develop immunity and resistance to certain influences.

One common approach to the study of new epidemics has been inspired by Ian Hacking's theories of dynamic nominalism (Hacking 1986, 1992) to think about the spread of diagnoses, categories and representations. The spread of diagnoses has been pointed out in relation to various mental problems such as autism (e.g. Grinker 2009; Seeberg and Christensen 2017), ADHD (e.g. Rasmussen and Meinert 2019; Timmi and Taylor 2003), depression (Brinkmann 2010) and PTSD (e.g. Fassin and Rechtman 2009; Young 1996). In Uganda, Whyte has pointed to the related phenomenon of awareness epidemics in relation to certain noncommunicable diseases such as diabetes and high blood pressure (Whyte 2012). This social constructionist perspective is well researched and documents that diagnostic and categorizing processes are contagious and play an active part in the configuration of epidemics. However, in this book we regard social contagion as more than social constructions that create epidemics of awareness, definition and discovery. We are interested in (social) contagion as intersubjective processes of influence and affection that are intertwined into epidemic configurations.

Configuring

We propose the analytical concept of configuring – employing the present progressive grammatical form to emphasize that a *process* is involved – in an attempt to form a framework for describing the figures and con-figures that create epidemic processes of biosocial contagion. As mentioned earlier, we build upon Rosenberg's description of configuration theories. Rosenberg describes and contrasts configuration explanations as an empirical and historical phenomenon that was common before contamination explanations became dominant with ideas about infection and microbiological contagion. Configuration theories, writes Rosenberg, typically explained epidemic disease as something that was caused by a disturbance of the social order, with health described as a balanced and integrated relation between human and environment (Rosenberg 1992: 295). We have suggested the term configuring as an analytical concept to describe dynamics that collaborate when social contagion happens (Seeberg and Meinert 2015). Configuring can be regarded as a form of contextualization (Seeberg and Christensen 2017). But whereas a context analysis is potentially endless (Dilley 1999), configuration analysis is an attempt to foreground certain figures and relations and their influence.

An epidemic is an expression of a specific configuration of various forms of social contagion and contamination, as well as other biosocial and material processes that happen over time. Specific epidemic configurations often contain several diseases and assemblages of problems simultaneously, and are therefore syndemic (Singer and Clair 2003). Epidemic configuring is dynamic in that problems and diagnoses change according to which phenomena, actors, institutions, practices and material conditions are involved (Williams and Meinert 2017). Diagnostic categories and biological and social phenomena of very different kinds (e.g. PTSD, spirits, viruses, social media) can all play a part in specific configurations. But configuration analysis can also be applied to understand transformations of epidemics when an epidemic disease develops antimicrobial resistance (Seeberg 2020).

We use the concept of configuring in order to achieve a broader understanding of (social) contagion and epidemics that reaches beyond causal and essentialist explanations (Seeberg, Roepstorff and Meinert 2020) as well as purely social constructionist models. Thinking in terms of configuration involves epistemological reconceptualization, with causal relations between various factors and units being supplemented by heuristic tools to explore a phenomenon. This perspective involves an epistemological shift from a correspondence theory about knowledge in which concepts work as mirrors of reality (Rorty 1980), to a pragmatic, testing and uncertain epistemology in which concepts are tried out as working hypotheses (Whyte 1997). In these contagious processes, local epistemologies, perceptions, assumptions, fears and apprehensions appear. Ideas about well-being that are historically grown, culturally specific and intersubjective in nature are all part of configuring processes.

In epidemiology, one effective way of thinking about processes influencing epidemics is in terms of disease agents, confounding factors and outcomes, and epidemiological analyses tend to single out specific agents and factors in lifestyles or life conditions as important for epidemic outcome. Policy approaches to the epidemics of non-infectious diseases have largely focused on lifestyle – understood as behaviour deemed risky in relation to specific conditions such as diabetes, lung cancer or obesity. Whereas these approaches focusing on lifestyle have no doubt been extremely important with a view to identifying specific dangerous practices, they have also been criticized for being behaviouristic, individualistic and mechanical (Coreil et al. 1985). Several Foucauldian analyses have pointed to the problematic promotion of prevention and treatment regimes, that seek to discipline the self (Petersen and Lupton 1996) and medicalize life itself (Rose 2007), whereas health issues often have to do with broader life conditions beyond individual lifestyle choices. Labelling certain illnesses as 'lifestyle diseases' can be thoroughly misleading (Seeberg and Meinert 2015). But in Weber's original framework, lifestyle was intimately linked to life conditions, through the concepts of *Lebensstil* (style of life), *Lebensführung* (conduct of life) and *Lebenschancen* (life chances). Life chances were conceived in socioeconomic terms (Weber 1999 (1922): 709–10) and linked to concepts such as class, whereas the first two concepts were linked to choice (Seeberg and Meinert 2015: 58). In our conception of configuring contagion, we are inspired by Weber's broad, sociological way of defining influence in our attempt to expand more narrow epidemiological definitions of agents, factors and outcomes.

We find the thinking of Singer and colleagues about syndemics useful for understanding how processes in which diseases or coinfections are intertwined reinforce each other at both biological and societal levels (Singer 2009; Singer and Clair 2003). Syndemic scholars have considered how infectious diseases create co-morbidity, and also how these and other diseases and conditions are intertwined with economic and social conditions as well as with ecological and environmental factors in what Singer defines as eco-syndemics (Singer 2012). Our thinking about configuring is in line with this school of thought, which reminds us that diseases are seldom separate units, but are interwoven phenomena in which life conditions and health problems are combined. This book's distinct contribution with the concept of configuring contagion highlights *the process of how* this interweaving and spreading happens in everyday lives, in networks of friends, family and social groups, under specific political and socioeconomic conditions, with an eye to how materialities and local epistemologies play into these processes.

The Contributions

The chapters in this book are based on contemporary ethnographic studies from the global north and south that develop critical theoretical reflections about the dynamics of configuring contagion in global health. The chapters are based on empirical material from Denmark, India, Indonesia, Niger, Oceania, Uganda, the USA and Latin America. The chapters will appeal in particular to anthropologists and other scholars within the social sciences and humanities with an interest in epidemics, as well as psychologists, psychiatrists and global health specialists interested in cultural health studies. The insights developed in this volume cut across disciplines with the intention of exploring how specific contexts, cases and diseases dynamically co-configure contagion.

Each chapter focuses on the configuring of contagion in relation to a specific disease, condition or social phenomenon, including suicide, autism, ADHD, trauma, spirits, abortion, obesity, porn addiction, Zika virus and drug-resistant tuberculosis. The chapters develop a range of different theoretical approaches to understand the configuration of contagion, and they engage with local perceptions of, fears of and words for contagion or polluting and contaminating substances, as well as local ideas about processes of configuring biological problems and social contexts. The chapters highlight the fact that contagion and configuration theories are not merely analyses that are externally imposed by the authors, but are shaped locally by historically specific and socially and ecologically attuned intersubjectivities. The chapters are developed from a selection of papers presented at a symposium on configuring contagion in biosocial epidemics organized by the Epicenter (the Centre for Cultural Epidemics) at Aarhus University in 2017.

The first two chapters of the book focus on suicide and its social configuration. Susan Reynolds Whyte and Henry Oboke write about gender discrepancies in completed suicides in northern Uganda. Based on archival material and contemporary data, they show that the gender discrepancy in this area has increased, with far more men than women committing suicide. The authors consider changing configurations of gender relations within families and between partners, and how masculinity has been challenged by war, encampment, disease, alcohol and poverty. Changes in gender configurations are related to broader patterns in political economy. Whyte and Oboke are not arguing for a single cause of the spread of suicide among men. Instead, they examine experience-near accounts in the context of these wider transformations in order to explore how contagious and contaminating affect relates to shifting configurations. Men talked about being bitter and angry because they felt they were not properly recognized and respected. The authors point out that configuring is also an endeavour undertaken by their interlocutors, who relate specific suicides to gender conflicts and failed filiation to fathers.

Edward Lowe's chapter draws on recent research on how the suicide problem is socially and experientially configured in the region of Oceania, particularly in Chuuk Lagoon. The chapter begins by presenting the way in which suicide cases are used in publicly mediated accounts as a metaphor for troubles associated with modernization and globalization, and the potential harm that these two processes cause in local indigenous populations. It then contrasts these generalizing epidemic readings of suicide to the way suicide is configured through lived experience as an endemic social practice in Chuuk and elsewhere in the region. One of the key points of focus in Lowe's ethnographic material is how suicide can grow out of a larger set of practices that aim to restore relational harmony and balance in the aftermath of a sudden breakdown in key social relationships. Lowe contrasts this endemic reading of suicide in Oceania with the way suicide is understood in the specialist literature in the United States, where suicide is regarded as a way to end painful internal psychological suffering connected to disruptions in a person's autobiographic self-making. In the concluding section, Lowe discusses how suicide both as discursive metaphor and as a phenomenon in lived experience can be understood as varieties of what Heidegger called presences that become manifest out of the larger, dynamic lifeworld, as well as discussing the implications of this insight for the study of biosocial epidemics.

Cheryl Mattingly and Stephanie Keeney Parks take us into the world of autism and incarceration in the African American community. They take up the idea of syndemics by considering the configuration of intellectual difference (autism) and the rapid rise of incarceration in many minority communities within the United States. Mattingly and Keeney Parks consider autism as a mental health classification that has taken on epidemic proportions, as it intersects with the epidemic of mass imprisonment within the African American community. The authors explore how African Americans employ local epistemologies to conceptualize the interconnection between the two phenomena. More specifically, they explore how African American parents of boys at risk of an ASD diagnosis in particular *respond* to the threat of this syndemic and the inoculating strategies they employ as they try to protect their boys from the life-threatening spectre of a life of unemployment and potential incarceration. The parents feel haunted by their future prospects. In their chapter, Mattingly and Keeney Parks draw on hauntology perspectives to think not just historically, but in terms of the return of phantasmal forms from buried pasts.

Lone Grøn focuses on the configuration of biosocial affection in the obesity epidemic in Denmark by exploring relatedness maps drawn by Danish families in which obesity has run for generations. Building on earlier work (Grøn 2017), where she suggests 'affection' as a phenomenological theory of social contagion that is characterized by indeterminacy and intersubjectivity, Grøn adds two further features. Firstly, the family experiences of contagion highlight affection as mutuality, as love, as belonging which is, however, both nourishing and poisonous, making contagion as affection especially haunting. Furthermore, the affective ties do not adhere to distinctions between what is biological and what is social, but emerge between material, biological, psychological, cultural, social and historical processes. Secondly, the configuration of diverse affections is specific and particular, which leads to different kinds of obesity, not only between families, but also within them. Obesity thus appears not as a monolithic category, but as obesities in the plural. Grøn argues that the notion of affection challenges prominent ideas about individual lifestyle and linear and demarcated causal pathways, which characterize contemporary debates and interventions as well as epidemiological approaches to obesity. The chapter presents instead an experience-near and anthropological approach that takes seriously the fact that academically demarcated territories between disciplines – and between individuals, others and the world – might not be helpful for understanding how obesity spreads.

While trauma may be seen to run in the family, like obesity, it can also affect much larger collectives in complex configurations. Jesse Hession Grayman, Mary-Jo DelVecchio Good and Byron Good explore changing social configurations of trauma in post-conflict, post-tsunami Aceh in Indonesia. This chapter interrogates the observation that a trauma triggered by conflict and/or a tsunami and experienced by the majority of Aceh's population reduced the stigma of mental illness, by reframing a 'fear of the other' (a contagion and confusion reaction to mental illness) as recognizable and deserving of compassion. High affect was associated with both the conflict and the tsunami, and the emotional intensity fed earnest approaches to reach out to treat those suffering from both disasters. This affective dimension is particularly powerful in energizing new ways of thinking about the mentally ill. Particularly notable is a professionalized willingness to confront the enormous challenges in caring for the seriously mentally ill, and to confront remainders of trauma embedded in historical events.

Lars Williams and Lotte Meinert discuss an extended case of trauma and spirit affliction after the war in northern Uganda to explore the configuration of affliction in a specific life, family and situation. They argue that being afflicted with trauma or spirits is a way of being 'touched' and contaminated by violence and death.

However, the experience is also configured as trauma and spirit affliction by psychotropic medication in the hospital, by local healers, and by prayer in church. In this way, contagious and contaminating elements from a legacy of violence con-figure – give figure to – afflictions of spirits and trauma. The authors describe how multiple treatment options for mental illness contribute to the configuration. When people combine different treatment options, the ways in which illness is expressed are transformed and configured through different paths of recovery. There is a market of healing with churches, NGOs, hospitals and traditional healers offering their services and tapping into each other as people travel through them in search of relief from their disorders.

Adeline Masquelier, Abouzeidi Maidouka Dillé and Ly Amadou H. Belko consider the relational dimensions of Nigerien girls' spirit possession as affliction through the analytical prism of contagion. By taking spirit possession and haunting to be a form of circulating affliction rather than individual resistance or somatization, or a way of dealing with conflict, Masquelier, Dillé and Belko consider schoolgirls' perceived susceptibility to others. They draw on the model of contagion elaborated by Gabriel Tarde to account for the rapid spread of ideas, fashions, technologies and crimes across a population. Through a focus on imitation – the ability to affect and be affected, consciously and unconsciously, by others – the authors highlight the extraordinary 'magnetic' power people can exert over each other in interactions. The authors argue that the mass possession of Nigerien schoolgirls indicates the way in which people incorporate others into themselves and are themselves embodied in others – a process that can be described as a contagion without contact.

Haunting may also be configured through internet-mediated fantasies and images, as shown in Doug Hollan's chapter on internet porn. He reflects on his meeting, as a therapist, with men who – although initially complaining about things such as depression, anxiety and various family and social problems – eventually shared their viewing of internet porn and the impact this had on their social, emotional and erotic lives. The chapter explores how contamination by sexual images and fantasies is configured and shaped by both social and personal factors. Hollan examines the role that culture, technology and institutions play in suppressing, articulating, exploiting or denying human fantasy and imaginative thought, and in turn, how the protean and creative aspects of human fantasies feed into and transform the sexual images currently available on the internet. The contamination the men felt when encountering sexual images on the internet affected them in different and non-transparent ways, depending on the history and development of their sexual and erotic lives.

Social contagion may seep through international and government bodies in ways that worsen the health outcomes of an unfolding epidemic. Lynn Morgan has studied the management of the outbreak of Zika virus in Latin America that started in 2015. Health agencies responded with education and prevention campaigns focused mainly on mosquito control and travel advice. Conspicuously absent from US and international Zika control campaigns was any attention to the need for contraceptives or prenatal screening, and nor did campaigns inform women about pregnancy termination options even in places where this was legal. By amplifying only certain kinds of knowledge, the authorities were complicit in producing ignorance and extending the suffering. This chapter argues that the configurations of contagion surrounding the Zika epidemic in Latin America reveal a widespread pattern of reproductive governance that relies on discrimination, stigma, secrecy and political cowardice. Meanwhile, as of 9 February 2017, 2,700 children in the western hemisphere had been confirmed with a congenital syndrome associated with Zika virus.

The configuration of contagion of tuberculosis (TB) has established it as the 'quintessential social disease' (Cervantes 2016) due to its preference for the socially disadvantaged and the stigmatization it attracts. It is perhaps less obvious that its transition to increasingly drug-resistant forms itself constitutes a form of biosocial contagion. In their chapter, Jens Seeberg, Bijayalaxmi Rautaray and Shyama Mohapatra explore drug resistance as a product of particular patterns of interaction between microbes, medicines and humans. Their analysis focuses on frictions experienced in the lives of people infected with drug-resistant TB in India as seen through the figures of Pharmacon, Regimen, Regula, Clinic and Oikonomia. Seeing these figures as production sites of resistance adds a new angle to the discussion of biosocial relations of production (Palsson 2016) in the field of tuberculosis. While infection with DRTB places the people affected in a situation of extreme vulnerability, individual life stories point to the mutuality of resistance and vulnerability. Actions of opposition, rejection and activism partially shape the configuration of the DRTB syndemic in its locality, pointing to resistance in vulnerability as much as vulnerability in resistance.

The volume concludes with an afterword by Byron Good reflecting on how the lens of configuring contagion may contribute to the understanding of very different kinds of biosocial epidemics and their mitigation.

Lotte Meinert
Professor, Department of Anthropology
Aarhus University, Denmark.

Jens Seeberg
Professor, Department of Anthropology
Aarhus University, Denmark.

Notes

1. See https://www.who.int/news-room/fact-sheets/detail/noncommunicable-diseases. Accessed 1 June 2020.
2. https://www.cdc.gov/csels/dsepd/ss1978/lesson1/section11.html. Accessed 14 June 2021.
3. Gabriel Tarde's work is often opposed to Durkheim's owing to his idea that the whole is always less than the sum of its parts; but here we are particularly interested in his ideas about imitation as a basic form of sociality with a view to thinking about how we might conceive of contagion as social influence.

References

Adjaye-Gbewonyo, K., and M. Vaughan. 2019. 'Reframing NCDs? An Analysis of Current Debates', *Global Health Action* 12(1).

Bateson, G. [1972] 2000. *Steps to an Ecology of Mind: Collected Essays in Anthropology, Psychiatry, Evolution, and Epistemology*. Chicago: Chicago University Press.

Boero, Nathalie. 2007. 'All the News That's Fat to Print: The American "Obesity Epidemic" and the Media', *Qualitative Sociology* 30(1): 41–60.

Blundell, H.J., and P. Hine. 2018. 'Non-Communicable Diseases: Ditch the Label and Recapture Public Awareness', *International Health* 11(1): 5–6.

Brinkmann, Svend (ed.). 2010. *Det Diagnosticerede Liv. Sygdom uden Grænser*. Aarhus: Klim.
Cervantes, Jorge. 2016. 'Tuberculosis. Digging Deep in the Soul of Humanity', *Respiratory Medicine* 119: 20–22. https://doi.org/10.1016/j.rmed.2016.08.009.
Coleman, Mischa, and Mason Littlejohn 2019. 'Health and Climate Change in Australia and the Asia Pacific Region: From Townsville to Tuvalu', Global Health Alliance Australia. Retrieved 9 July from http://glham.org/wp-content/uploads/GLHAA_TownsvilleTuvalu-08.pdf.
Coreil, J., J.S. Levin and E.G. Jaco. 1985. 'Life Style: An Emergent Concept in the Sociomedical Sciences', *Culture, Medicine and Psychiatry* 9(4): 423–437.
Dilley, Roy. 1999. 'Introduction. The Problem of Context', in R. Dilley (ed.), *The Problem of Context*. New York: Berghahn Books, pp. 1–46.
Eigen, Manfred, John McCaskill and Peter Schuster. 1989. 'The Molecular Quasi-Species', *Advances in Chemical Physisc* 75: 149–263.
Fainzang, Sylvie. 1996. 'Alcoholism, a Contagious Disease: A Contribution towards an Anthropological Definition of Contagion', *Culture, Medicine and Psychiatry* 20: 473–87.
Fassin, Didier, and Richard Rechtman. 2009. *The Empire of Trauma: An Inquiry into the Condition of Victimhood*. Princeton, NJ: Princeton University Press.
Folmann, Birgitte. 2017. 'The Social Contagion of Aspirations: On the Happiness of Having a "Life Style"', *Tidsskrift for Forskning i Sygdom og Samfund* 26: 41–61.
Garcia, Angela. 2014. 'Regeneration: Love Drugs, and the Making of Hispano Inheritance', *Social Anthropology* 22(2): 200–12.
Garcia, Angela. 2019. 'Fragments of Relatedness: Writing, Archiving, and the Vicissitudes of Kinship', *Ethnos* 85(4): 717–29. doi:10.1080/00141844.2019.1645190.
Good, Byron J. 2015. 'Haunted by Aceh: Specters of Violence in Post-Suharto Indonesia', in Devon E. Hinton and Alexander L. Hinton (eds), *Genocide and Mass Violence: Memory, Symptom, and Recovery*. Cambridge: Cambridge University Press, pp. 58–82.
Grinker, Roy Richard. 2009. *Isabel's World: Autism and the Making of a Modern Epidemic*. Thriplow: Icon.
Grøn, Lone. 2017. 'The Weight of the Family: Communicability as Alien Affection in Danish Family Histories and Experiences of Obesity', *Ethos* 45(2): 182–98.
Grøn, Lone. 2019. 'Cutting/Belonging. Sameness and Difference in the Lived Experience of Obesity and Kinship in Denmark', *Ethnos* 85(4): 679–95. doi: 10.1080/00141844.2019.1626465.
Grøn, Lone, and Lotte Meinert. 2017. 'Social Contagion and Cultural Epidemics: Phenomenological and "Experience-Near" Explorations', *Ethos* 45(2): 165–81.
Hacking, Ian. 1986. 'Making Up People', in T. Heller, M. Sosna and D. Wellberry (eds), *Reconstructing Individualism*. Palo Alto, CA: Stanford University Press, pp. 222–36.

Hacking, Ian. 1992. 'World-Making by Kind-Making: Child Abuse for Example', in M. Douglas and D. Hull (eds), *How Classification Works*. Edinburgh: Edinburgh University Press, pp. 180–238.

Han, Clara, and Andrew Brandel. 2019. 'Genres of Witnessing: Narrative, Violence, Generations', *Ethnos* 85(4): 629–46. doi:10.1080/00141844.2019.1630466.

Hollan, Douglas. 2017. 'Dreamscapes of Intimacy and Isolation: Shadows of Contagion and Immunity', *Ethos* 45(2): 216–31. doi:10.1111/etho.12166.

Ingold, Tim. 2013. 'Ensembles of Biosocial Relations', in Tim Ingold and Gisli Palsson (eds), *Biosocial Becomings: Integrating Social and Biological Anthropology*. Cambridge: Cambridge University Press, pp. 22–41.

Kuan, Teresa. 2019. 'Feelings Run in the Family: Kin Therapeutics and the Configuration of Cause in China', *Ethnos* 85(4): 696–716. doi:10.1080/00141844.2019.1634614.

Lawlor, M.C., and O. Solomon. 2017. 'A Phenomenological Approach to the Cultivation of Expertise: Emergent Understandings of Autism', *Ethos* 45(2): 232–49. doi:10.1111/etho.12162.

Livingston, Julie. 2020. 'When Sickness Comes in Multiples: Co-morbidity in Botswana', in Jens Seeberg, Andreas Roepstorff and Lotte Meinert (eds), *Biosocial Worlds: Anthropology of Health Environments beyond Determinism*. London: UCL Press, https://www.uclpress.co.uk/products/154838.

Lowe, Celia. 2010. 'Viral Clouds: Becoming H5N1 in Indonesia', *Cultural Anthropology* 25(4): 625–49.

Maji, Avijit, Tushar Choudhari and M.B. Sushma. 2020. 'Implication of Repatriating Migrant Workers on COVID-19 Spread and Transportation Requirements', *Transportation Research Interdisciplinary Perspectives* 7:100187. https://doi.org/10.1016/j.trip.2020.100187.

Martin, P., and E. Martin-Granel. 2006. '2,500-Year Evolution of the Term Epidemic', *Emerging Infectious Diseases* 12(6): 976–80.

Matthews, P.C. 1968. 'Epidemic Self-Injury in an Adolescent Unit', *International Journal of Social Psychiatry* 14: 125–33.

Mattingly, Cheryl. 2017. 'Autism and the Ethics of Care: A Phenomenological Investigation into the Contagion of Nothing', *Ethos* 45(2): 250–70. doi:10.1111/etho.12164.

Meinert, Lotte. 2019. 'Haunted Families after the War in Uganda: Doubt as Polyvalent Critique', *Ethnos* 85(4): 595–611. doi:10.1080/00141844.2019.1629981.

Meinert, Lotte, and Lone Grøn. 2019. '"It Runs in the Family": Exploring Contagious Kinship Connections', *Ethnos* 85(4): 581–94. doi:10.1080/00141844.2019.1640759.

Meinert, Lotte, and Jens Seeberg. 2008. 'Epidemier: Introduktion', *Tidsskrift for Forskning i Sygdom og Samfund* 8: 5–9.

Meinert, Lotte, and Susan R. Whyte. 2017. 'These Things Continue: Violence as Contamination in Everyday Life after War in Northern Uganda', *Ethos* 45(2): 271–86. doi:10.1111/etho.12161.

Moffat, Tina. 2010. 'The Childhood Obesity Epidemic: Health Crisis or Social Construction?', *Medical Anthropology Quarterly* 24(1): 1–21.

Napier, A. David. 2013. 'A New Sociobiology: Immunity, Alterity, and the Social Repertoire', *Cambridge Anthropology* 31(2): 20–43.

Nielsen, Jeanette Lykkegaard. 2017. 'Alkohol og Relationalitet: Social Smitte som Animistisk Fænomen i Sibirien', *Tidsskrift for Forskning i Sygdom og Samfund* 26: 109–26.

Oboke, Henry, and Susan Reynolds Whyte. 2019. 'Anger and Bitter Hearts: The Spread of Suicide in Northern Ugandan Families', *Ethnos* 85(4): 612–28. doi:10.1080/00141844.2019.1629982.

Palsson, Gisli. 2016. *Nature, Culture and Society: Anthropological Perspectives on Life*. Cambridge: Cambridge University Press.

Pernick, M.S. 2002. 'Contagion and Culture', *American Literary History* 14(4): 858–65.

Petersen, Alan, and Deborah Lupton. 1996. *The New Public Health: Health and Self in the Age of Risk*. Thousand Oaks, CA: Sage.

Rasmussen, Gitte, and Lotte Meinert. 2019. 'ADHD – En Tidstypisk Tidsforstyrrelse?', *Tidsskrift for Forskning i Sygdom og Samfund* 30: 199–217.

Rorty, R. 1980. *Philosophy and the Mirror of Nature*. Vol. 401. Cambridge: Cambridge University Press.

Rosa, Hartmut. 2019. *Resonance: A Sociology of Our Relationship to the World*. Cambridge: Polity Press.

Rose, Nikolas. 2007. *The Politics of Life Itself: Biomedicine, Power, and Subjectivity in the Twenty-First Century*. Princeton, NJ: Princeton University Press.

Rosenberg, C.E. 1992. *Explaining Epidemics and Other Studies in the History of Medicine*. Cambridge: Cambridge University Press.

Scheper-Hughes, Nancy, and Margaret M. Lock. 1987. 'The Mindful Body: A Prolegomenon to Future Work in Medical Anthropology', *Medical Anthropology Quarterly* 1(1): 6–41.

Seeberg, Jens. 2019. 'Fear of Drug-Resistant Tuberculosis as Social Contagion', *Ethnos* 85(4): 665–78. doi:10.1080/00141844.2019.1634615.

Seeberg, Jens. 2020. 'Biosocial Dynamics of Multidrug-Resistant Tuberculosis: A Bacterial Perspective', in Jens Seeberg, Andreas Roepstorff and Lotte Meinert (eds), *Biosocial Worlds: Anthropology of Health Environments beyond Determinism*. London: UCL Press, pp. 124–45.

Seeberg, Jens, and Fie Lund Christensen. 2017. 'Configuring the Autism Epidemic: Why Are So Few Girls Diagnosed?', *Tidsskrift for Forskning i Sygdom og Samfund* 14(26): 127–44.

Seeberg, Jens, and Lotte Meinert. 2015. 'Can Epidemics Be Non-Communicable? Reflections on the Spread of "Non-Communicable" Diseases', *Medicine Anthropology Theory* 2(2): 54–71.

Seeberg Jens, Andreas Roepstorff and Lotte Meinert. 2020. 'Introduction: Biosocial Worlds', in Jens Seeberg, Andreas Roepstorff and Lotte Meinert (eds), *Biosocial Worlds: Anthropology of Health Environments beyond*

Determinism. London: UCL Press, pp. 1–14. https://www.uclpress.co.uk/products/154838.
Singer, Merrill. 2009. *Introduction to Syndemics: A Systems Approach to Public and Community Health*. San Francisco, CA: Jossey-Bass.
Singer, Merill, and Scott Clair. 2003. 'Syndemics and Public Health: Reconceptualizing Disease in Bio-Social Context', *Medical Anthropology Quarterly* 17(4): 423–41.
Singer, Merrill, Nicola Bulled and Bayla Ostrach. 2012. 'Syndemics and Human Health: Implications for Prevention and Intervention', *Annals of anthropological practice* 36(2): 205–211.
Singer, Merrill, et al. 2017. 'Syndemics and the Biosocial Conception of Health', *Lancet* 389(10072): 941–50.
Stevenson, Lisa. 2019. 'What There Is to Fear: Scenes of Worldmaking and Unmaking in the Aftermaths of Violence', *Ethnos* 85(4): 647–64. doi:10.1080/00141844.2019.1636843.
Stewart, Kathleen. 2007. *Ordinary Affect*. Durham, NC: Duke University Press.
Tarde, Gabriel de. 1903. *The Laws of Imitation*. New York: Henry Holt and Company.
Taylor, Charles. 1989. *The Sources of the Self: The Making of the Modern Identity*. Cambridge, MA: Harvard University Press.
Throop, C.J. 2017. 'Despairing Moods: Worldly Attunements and Permeable Personhood in Yap', *Ethos* 45(2): 199–215. doi:10.1111/etho.12163.
Timmi, Sami, and Eric Taylor. 2003. 'ADHD Is Best Understood as a Cultural Construct', *British Journal of Psychiatry* 184(1): 8–9.
Waldenfels, Bernhard. 2011. *Phenomenology of the Alien: Basic Concepts*. Evanston, IL: Northwestern University Press.
Weber, Max. 1999. 'Class, Status, Party' (1922), in H.H. Gerth and C.W. Mills (eds), *From Max Weber: Essays in Sociology*. New York: Oxford University Press.
Whyte, Susan Reynolds. 1997. *Questioning Misfortune: The Pragmatics of Uncertainty in Eastern Uganda*. Cambridge: Cambridge University Press.
Whyte, Susan Reynolds. 2012. 'Chronicity and Control: Framing Noncommunicable Diseases in Africa', *Anthropology and Medicine* 19(1): 63–74.
Williams, Lars, and Lotte Meinert. 2017. 'Traumer og Ånder efter Krig i Uganda: Konfigurationer af Vold og Behandling', *Tidsskrift for Forskning i Sygdom og Samfund* 26: 63–88.
Young, Allan. 1996. *The Harmony of Illusions: Inventing Post Traumatic Stress Disorder*. New Jersey: Princeton University Press.

Chapter 1
Gender Configurations and Suicide in Northern Uganda

Susan Reynolds Whyte and Henry Oboke

In northern Uganda, suicide runs in families through affect. Feelings of resentment, betrayal and humiliation take hold within kin relations, embittering hearts and giving rise to the anger that makes people take their own lives. Archival material from 1925 to 1954 reveals that this is an old pattern, for which there are many local terms and modes of expression. What has changed is the gender pattern of suicide. Data assembled between 2014 and 2016 show that gender discrepancies in completed suicides have increased, with far more men than women killing themselves today. From interviews with bereaved families and people who attempted suicide, together with records kept by village counsellors, we gathered accounts of challenged masculinity exacerbated by war, encampment, disease, alcohol and poverty. The decline in formal marriage and increase in children of single mothers might seem to affect women's security most directly, but in some ways men feel these changes heavily. We heard many stories of men who were bitter and angry because they felt they were not properly recognized and respected. Changes in gender configurations are related to broader patterns in political economy; we are not arguing for a single cause of the spread of suicide among men. Instead, we examine experience-near accounts in the context of these wider transformations in order to explore how contagious and contaminating affect relates to shifting configurations. We emphasize that configuring is also an endeavour undertaken by our interlocutors, and we are alert to the ways in which they understand changes in gender relations that might be related to patterns of suicide.

**

Arriving at the home of a family that had lost a man – a son, husband and father – to suicide, we were taken directly to an overgrown place at the edge of the compound. Our hosts wanted to show us the charred stump of the tree from which Noah had hanged himself. It had been wet at that time when he died three years earlier, and they had not been able to burn the tree completely. But they planned to finish the work when they performed his last funeral rites; as they explained, it was not good to leave such material where some bad-hearted person might take a piece of it to use maliciously to cause another suicide.

The two of us, an anthropologist and a clinical psychologist, spent a long afternoon with that family, and heard first from Noah's mother and later from his wife Spora, accounts of what led up to his death. They coincided more or less, emphasizing a history of angry confrontations with several family members living in the large compound. The culmination was a violent fight with his wife. He beat her because he saw her at a neighbourhood dance, though he had not given her permission to leave home. He would not listen to her explanation that she was only bringing a crying baby left in her care to its mother at the nearby party. It enraged him that his own mother tried to protect his wife. His mother told us how she stopped him from beating his wife, saying, 'these days women are not quarrelled with like that'. He kicked and beat his mother and her sister, shouting: 'Why stop me from beating my wife whom I married? No one helped me pay bridewealth for her'. He disappeared, still angry. When his son looked for him in his house, he saw the bed tipped over and the mosquito net missing. It was his mother who finally found him hanging from the fateful tree at the edge of the compound, his feet almost touching the ground, having twisted the mosquito net as a rope. She told us how she started slapping his dangling body, asking, 'What are you doing here?'

Noah's wife and mother remembered other occasions when Noah had become very angry, sometimes when drunk, and threatened suicide. On one occasion he quarrelled bitterly with his mother's sister, when she accidently burned a hut; defending her daughter, his grandmother hurled at him a reminder that his father had never claimed him. Noah was born and grew up in the home of his mother, who was staying with her mother and another sister. Such a matrifocal household, composed of daughters and their children staying with mothers, did not correspond to the patrilineal virilocal ideal of Acholi gender organization, in which women stay in their husband's home so that children grow up with, and belong to, their fathers.

Then there were the running tensions between Noah and his wife Spora, when he took another wife whom he kept in town. Spora gave an example: 'He would come back from his second wife in town with dirty clothes for me to wash. I refused because he dirtied them on paths going to another woman'. In the accounts of both Noah's mother and his wife, another conflict had worried him and continued to cause them anxiety: the man who had inherited Noah's mother after her husband died was claiming their land and had already sold a portion of it.

The accounts of Noah's death pointed to gender conflicts: the immediate quarrels with his wife, but also earlier gender issues in that his mother and father did not live together and his father never recognized him. Heavy drinking and conflicts over resources contributed to Noah's anger and distress, but it is the gender discord that we wish to explore.

Noah's suicide was one of many that occurred in the Acholi sub-region of northern Uganda during the years of the war against the Lord's Resistance Army (LRA) from 1986 to 2006 and after. In particular, the period from 2012 to 2014, when people who had been interned in camps for the Internally Displaced had settled back into their rural homes, was marked by a wave of suicides that seemed to assume epidemic proportions. The national and local news media reported on the rising rates, attributed to trauma and depression after the war, the vengeful ghosts (*cen*) of those who were killed, poverty and alcoholism (e.g. Aber 2012; Akena and Kidega 2012; Owich 2016). Several of the newspaper articles identified domestic conflicts as immediate causes of male suicide. 'Joseph Bodo, the Dog-Dago village LC1 chairperson in Adilang sub-county, Agago district, says most of the cases stem from domestic violence [or quarrels], citing the example of a resident, who burnt to death after he set his hut ablaze, following a disagreement with his wife' (Aber 2012). In one case in Nwoya district, a woman had to seek police protection from neighbours who wanted to kill her in revenge for her husband's suicide. They held her responsible because the pair were on bad terms, with the husband accusing her of ill-treatment. This happened only a week after another man in the district killed himself after a 'domestic misunderstanding' (Owich 2014). Strikingly, those who commit suicide after 'domestic violence' or 'misunderstandings' are reported to be men.

In this chapter, we consider gender disparities in suicide as reported in other research from the Acholi sub-region and more generally in the literature on Africa. We use cases we ourselves assembled to analyse two themes: conflicts between partners; and children's paternal filiation. We then discuss the ways that the interlocutors themselves, in our study and in others, seem to understand the social dynamics of suicide. But first, we explain our methods and our use of the concept of configuration.

Now and Then

Our material on suicide in the Acholi sub-region comes from ethnographic interviews and from archival material. The background was Henry Oboke's PhD project, which involved training sixty-three lay village counsellors to document and try to prevent self-harm. We reviewed their statistical records of suicide incidents in their villages and the short descriptions in their notebooks. In 2015 and 2016, we interviewed six of them and they brought us to homes, such as that of Noah, where we were able to discuss seven relatively recent suicides. They also introduced us to four people who talked with us about their suicide attempts. Of these eleven cases, there were five in which we were able to talk to more than one family member. In Koro sub-county, we had a long discussion with the traditional chief (*rwot moo*), and on another day with his council of elders, about the very high number of suicides that had occurred there. Only this latter discussion was digitally recorded. All the others were captured in notes handwritten on the spot, expanded upon entry into a computer, and reviewed by both of us.

We were able to compare suicide in postwar Acholiland to earlier patterns, thanks to an archive at Boston University's African

Studies Library containing material assembled by anthropologist Paula Hirsch Foster between 1955 and 1959. Apparently Foster intended to contribute a chapter to Paul Bohannon's edited volume, *African Homicide and Suicide* (1967). She had followed his guidelines, examining inquest and court records for the period 1925–54. A careful ethnographer, proficient in Acholi, Foster left notes as well, including a transcription of an interview with the pedagogical and reflective Chief Jeremiah Ajwayo, whose wife had committed suicide. She never wrote her chapter for Bohannon's book, but photocopies of the painstakingly collected data, typed on creased and ragged onion-skin paper, have added a historical dimension to our considerations of suicide in Acholiland today.

Contamination and Configuration

In his book *Explaining Epidemics* (1992), the medical historian Charles Rosenberg distinguishes between contrasting, but often complementary views of how disease spreads. He uses the term *configuration* for 'a health-maintaining and health-constituting arrangement of climate, environment and communal life' (1992: 295). A disease extends its reach when such arrangements are disturbed, allowing a sickness to take hold. The term *contamination* he reserves for 'any event or agent that might subvert a health-maintaining configuration' (ibid.). A configuration is a system of relationships, a kind of ecology, that can be disturbed by a contaminating force.

The two modes of thinking about epidemics often go together and we can discern both in the material about suicide in Acholiland. As we have set out elsewhere (Oboke and Whyte 2019), we see contamination taking several forms as a factor in the spread of suicide. Suicide is said to be 'catching' through proximity, either through material contact (thus the need to destroy the tree from which Noah hanged himself) or through social connection (the idea that the ghost of a suicide may move others in the family to take their lives). It is also contagious through 'affective contamination' between intimates when indignation, resentment, humiliation, abuse and disrespect make hearts bitter (*cweer cwiny*) and give rise to the anger (*kiniga*) that can push a person to suicide. We examined these forms of contamination as 'agents' in Rosenberg's terms, setting out the ways in which one suicide is thought to lead to another and the ways in which feelings affect family members and create suicidal anger.

Here we turn to Rosenberg's other concept, that of configuration, in order to understand how changes in the arrangements of communal life, in the conditions of social interaction, might have opened the way for suicide to spread. Relying on the material assembled by Foster in late colonial times, we found continuities in the kinds of contamination alleged to be immediate agents of suicide. Notions of suicide running in families persist. Anger, humiliation, shame, bitterness and a sense of betrayal are as evident in our recent interviews as they were in the much terser entries in the inquest records. What has changed strikingly is the gender pattern of suicide, suggesting transformations in the configuration of gender relations. In Acholi communities, social harmony (*ber bedo* or staying well) is highly valued (Obika et al. 2018; Porter 2012). As Porter (2016) has shown, maintaining such harmony can mean that women accept male authority and sexual privilege, keeping quiet about men's aggression if open confrontation would disturb domestic and neighbourhood serenity. The ideals and practices that maintain social harmony are part of general configurations of gender relations; as those configurations change, or are contaminated, civility and harmony are disrupted.

The Predominance of Male Suicide

Globally, men commit suicide more frequently than women and the social construction of gender is clearly key to understanding this preponderance (Payne, Swami and Stanistreet 2008). The degree of disparity varies widely among regions and countries. For the African region, the World Health Organization (WHO) estimates that about twice as many men as women take their own lives (WHO 2019). Suicide statistics are difficult to compile accurately, especially in Africa, where suicide is a criminal offence in many countries. But even if records are insufficient, available figures give a general picture. Bohannon's project on suicide and homicide attempted a systematic registration of data from inquest and court records in the late colonial period. The Ugandan case studies showed a predominance of male suicides in those years, though not a massive one: 69 per cent of suicides among the Soga were by men; 61 per cent among the Nyoro; and 59 per cent among the Gisu (Bohannon [1960] 1967: 261). An examination of inquest records for approximately the same era in Nyasaland found that men killed themselves at an even higher rate: three times as frequently as women (Vaughan 2010: 395).

These studies of older patterns found that masculinity issues were commonly reported as reasons for suicide.

> Impotence, or fear of it, is a constant theme in many African societies, which often leads to suicide ... there are cases of men who committed suicide when their domestic situation was threatened, by faulty social relationships, by disease, or by some other misfortune. (Bohannon [1960] 1967: 262)

> Men's anger at women and frustration at the poverty of their households emerges clearly from these accounts, but the fact that some men went on to kill themselves after these incidents reveals an additional dimension of anxiety about how their actions would be judged with their communities. (Vaughan 2010: 399)

More recent research from southern Africa confirms the predominance of male suicide. In his material on fifty-two suicides in Bushbuckridge, northeastern South Africa, Niehaus found that 75 per cent were male. He notes that while many studies of suicide acknowledge male social hegemony, they 'fail to explain why the dominant are more likely to commit suicide than the dominated' (Niehaus 2012: 329). In addressing this question, he draws on Moore's contrast between gender as 'constructed' and 'lived'. He suggests that men invest in an ideology of male dominance that is often thwarted in practice. In Bourdieu's terms, they suffer symbolic violence because they are humiliated by failure to dominate. Although he does not write of suicide as 'epidemic', we might consider Niehaus's exposition in Rosenberg's terms. Niehaus describes earlier configurations of gender relations that were more congruent with the ideal of male dominance: men were migrant labourers and women were dependent on their wages. De-industrialization and the AIDS epidemic were the contaminants that undermined that configuration. Niehaus provides an overview of these as historical facts. But he also touches on another point: the reflections on gender that were provoked by particular suicides.

Reflectivity is a central theme in Livingston's (2009) consideration of suicide in Botswana. She identifies several different suicide narratives, all of which relate the rising rate of suicide, and particularly of male suicide, to recent developments in Botswana society. She too discusses the paradox that more men kill themselves, despite their political, economic and social power. And she points to another similar puzzle: increasingly, middle-class people are committing suicide rather than those most affected by poverty and lack of opportunity. Male anger and failed expectations figure in her account, sometimes playing out in a scenario in which men kill their partners and then turn their aggression on themselves.

Our material from northern Uganda comes from two different sources – archival records and recent interviews – with an interval of more than sixty years. Nevertheless, we think it makes a clear point. The gender incidence of suicide has changed radically, with men now taking their own lives far more frequently than women.[1] Paula Hirsch Foster retrieved information on 122 suicides in Gulu district from inquest records between 1925 and 1954. There were sixty-two men and sixty women; thus the gender ratio was almost 1:1. For 2015 and 2016, Henry's lay counsellors recorded suicides in the twelve sub-counties of old Gulu district. There were eighty-five men and twenty-five women, giving a female to male ratio of 1:3.4. Another study, carried out by a Norwegian-Ugandan team while people were still interned in IDP camps, found a similarly skewed ratio of 1:4.4 (Kizza et al. 2012b: 697). The predominance of male suicide in Acholiland has been attributed to the experience of war and internment, which made it difficult for men to realize existing ideals of masculinity.

Chris Dolan carried out fieldwork in IDP camps primarily from 1998 to 2000 while the war was ongoing, and wrote a comprehensive description of the psychological and social consequences of the conflict. He asserted that men experienced a loss of domestic and political power and suffered humiliation because they were unable to achieve the hegemonic model of masculinity (see Connell and Messerschmidt 2005) by creating, providing for and protecting a family (Dolan 2009: 205). He considered suicide, impotence and alcohol abuse to be symptoms of this.

Whereas explanations for over-drinking embrace the loss of masculinity in the widest sense of a loss of social power and control, explanations given for men's suicides are much more directly focused on their unsatisfactory relations with women ... Twelve of the fifteen cases were directly attributed to a failure to achieve the hegemonic model of marriage and of control over women. (Dolan 2009: 207–8)

Gender relations were further problematic because of the high prevalence of HIV/AIDS, for which no treatment was available at that time.

A few years after Dolan's research, Kizza and colleagues undertook a careful psychological autopsy study of seventeen male suicides in 2007–8, interviewing two to five family members for each case. They found, as did we, that mental illness played almost no role in relatives' understanding of a suicide. Intimate others explained the circumstances of death in ways that the researchers reduced to a few themes: lost dignity and social value; no hope for the family's future; and overwhelming family responsibility. Mindful of the social and cultural factors that might lead to these negative feelings, they considered gender values in Acholi society, and the changes in life conditions and gender expectations that might explain differences in male and female suicide patterns. 'The effects and after-effects of war challenged the men's ability to be "men", causing identity or existential crises for many' (Kizza et al. 2012b: 710). For women too, the war was key: 'We contend that power struggles between husbands and wives brought about by the changes in gender roles following the protracted armed conflict/war, was [sic] crucial in the young women's perception of lost control in life in Northern Uganda' (Kizza et al. 2012c: 9).

Changes in gender relations can be traced back to colonial times. Girling, who did fieldwork in 1949–50, reported that adultery and divorce were on the rise, as was the status of women. Husbands who beat their wives were liable to fines and imprisonment by the government chiefs (Girling 1960: 194–95). Foster, working a few years after Girling, also found that men felt challenged by women's increasing autonomy (Lagace 2014). Still, bridewealth was being paid in the late colonial period and all women married formally at some point, even if they changed partners occasionally.

Foster's suicide records contain many examples of deaths attributed to gender conflicts, but they were of a different nature than those reported in recent times.

> 15 March 1948. Ludya Auulu, age 35, hanged herself from the roof beam of her house. The coroner stated: she had incurred her husband's disapproval because for 13 years she failed to bear any children. The day before, her husband had refused her permission to visit Gulu.

> 13 October 1948. Paiyo, age 27, hanged herself in her house. Her husband stated: 'She was the wife of my dead brother, and I wanted her to be my wife. She refused and went with another man, not our clan. I went to the Jago [government chief] who ordered her to be my wife. I called the villagers and asked her if she agrees. She did. I killed a goat as is custom, when I brought her here and she killed herself while we were drinking'.

> 10 January 1949. Olanya Lulyel, age 30, hung himself in the bush. It is alleged that he killed himself because he was unable to marry and was still a bachelor.

> 15 September 1949. Kag, age 27, hanged herself from a tree. It is alleged that the woman was angry because her husband did not want to complete her dowry since 1936.

> 4 January 1952. Timalo Onyero, age 22, hanged himself from a tree in the bush. Witnesses stated: he killed himself after his wife's father came and took away his wife for insufficient dowry.

The gender conflicts mentioned in the old inquest records suggested that women were thought to kill themselves as a rejection of male control and that both sexes were distraught by failure to achieve formalized marriage. That may have been changing already before the LRA war commenced in 1986. But the loss of all livestock and the long internment in the IDP camps, where it was almost impossible to earn money, put a complete stop to the payment of bridewealth: 'it is the denial of marriage, that core concept of adult masculinity, which is at the heart of many frustrations' (Dolan 2009: 211). While formal marriage through the exchange of marriage dues and the ritual involvement of both families is declining all over the country, the transition has been especially abrupt in the areas of the north affected by the war and internment.

Gender Conflicts

Our own investigations, which took place seven years after most people left the camps and returned to their rural homes, found a continuation of themes identified by Dolan, Kizza and colleagues. In almost all of the ten cases of male suicides or attempts that we discussed, men seemed to feel betrayal, humiliation and disrespect in connection with conflicts between partners. In several cases, women 'stubbornly' or angrily refused to accept men's authority to do as they liked. The closure of the camps, phasing out of humanitarian food rations and resumption of farming brought certain reconfigurations of partner conflict. Families were again able to accumulate a few resources and some men were even able to make bridewealth payments. Yet resources were still scarce; the reports about suicides mentioned conflicts between partners over livestock, money and material possessions.

Rose, a frail sickly woman, fluently told the story of the suicide of her husband's brother Samuel. By that time, her own husband, a soldier posted to Moroto, had already died and she was inherited by another of her husband's brothers. They all stayed in one large compound together with her mother-in-law and the children. The flue for drying tobacco indicated that they had a cash crop and were not as desperately poor as many others. Rose said that Samuel had a bitter heart (*cwee cwinyi*) because every year after harvest his wife took things back to her natal home. In 2010 the wife was due to receive her shares from two savings groups (*boli cup*) of which she was a member. Evidently an enterprising woman, she had plans to buy a cow with the money. When her husband and others in the family went to a funeral in Gulu, she packed everything in the house but one bedsheet and went to her own family, leaving their three children with her mother-in-law. Samuel was upset, and sold a goat ostensibly to get money to follow his wife. But instead, he used the money to buy clothes and to drink. His lineage brothers brought him back from the bar dead drunk and disciplined him by giving him ten strokes with a stick in front of his mother. Angry and humiliated, he told his brothers to prepare a grave for the next day. Still drunk, he downed a bottle of Ambush insecticide. They rushed him to hospital but he died there. After his death, his wife, whom he had married properly, returned and was inherited by his brother.

Both his sister-in-law Rose and his nephew living nearby emphasized Samuel's anger and resentment against his wife because she regularly stored crops with her own family after harvest and because she cleared the house of all their property while he was away. We did not hear the wife's side of the story but it could well be that she was trying to protect household resources from her husband's drinking. Certainly that pattern was identified by media reports about other suicides:

> At least ten local farmers in Nwoya district are known to have committed suicide after disagreeing with their spouses over the sale of farm harvests in the last one month alone. ... Mr. Patrick Okello Oryema, the District Chairman LCV ... explained that 'The problem is being fueled by men who are selling farm produce without the consent of their wives and wasting it on alcohol and extramarital affairs in busy trading centers'. (Owich 2014)

> Last week, 50-year-old Santo Adiri of Abole Village reportedly drank poison after a disagreement with his wife. Adiri had wanted to sell their maize in order to buy pigs and use part of the money for drinking alcohol, a move [to which] his wife objected. (Akena and Kidega 2012)

Samuel's wife may have been especially keen to hide the money she was to receive from her savings group, money she would have considered hers, not theirs.

Six years after Samuel's death and just a few months prior to our visit, Rose's eldest son Okumu tried to commit suicide, again after a marital conflict. With the help of his father's brothers, he had paid bridewealth for his first wife, mother to three of his children. In 2016, his younger second wife, with whom he had one child, was taken back to her home by her family because he had not paid for either the child or the wife. According to Rose, Okumu ordered the first wife to help care for the tobacco garden of the second wife while she was away. He was furious when she refused and he swallowed 100 capsules of amoxicillin that had been kept after visits to the health centre. She grabbed his throat and forced him to choke some of them out. According to Okumu himself, the disagreement was about money. Together with his father's brother, he had taken a payment to the home of his second wife. The first wife had misplaced some cash and thought Okumu had taken it to pay the family of the second wife. 'She thought the money was

Gender Configurations and Suicide in Northern Uganda

from her sweat. But it was mine. I explained how I got the money but she persisted so I could not tolerate.' Her quarrelling and the false accusation made his heart angry (*cwera cunya*) and drove him to swallow the pills. (She found her money later and apologized for blaming him.)[2]

Like his father's brother Samuel, Okumu had long running disagreements with his wife. In his case, part of the problem seems to have been her resentment of her co-wife. For both couples, tensions revolved around control of resources. What is striking is that the accounts position the men as driven to suicide when they cannot enforce their will upon their wives. These women did not accept male authority in the interest of social harmony; the configuration of gender relations was shifting.

Filiation of Children

The relations of children, particularly sons, to their fathers is of structural importance in a patrilineal society. Children should belong to their fathers' lineage and clan, but that requires that he recognize them by making a payment to the family of their mother. If he does not marry her properly with bridewealth, he should at least offer *luk*, a prestation that acknowledges his paternity. It has long been the case that women sometimes bore children without marrying the father and that sons grew up in their maternal home. If no *luk* payment was made, such children were absorbed in their mother's family. But this seems to have emerged as a problem of great concern after people left the camps. Conflicts over access to land meant that some families tried to enforce a kind of 'patrilineal fundamentalism' that would exclude the sons of daughters and sisters from their mothers' homes and land (Whyte et al. 2013: 294). The commonly discussed 'nephew problem' referred to sons of sisters, not sons of brothers. Here too configurations of gender relations changed. Partly, there were more children without socially recognized fathers because of the decline of formal marriage. But even children born before the war whose paternity was not acknowledged were now seen as a problem in their mothers' homes. The issue of the filiation of children, particularly sons, was evident in several of the situations we examined.

Susan Reynolds Whyte and Henry Oboke

One afternoon in October 2016, we sat in the large, well-kept compound of 56-year-old Augustino, a thin, unhappy-looking man. His ragged yellow t-shirt with the letters NRM, for the ruling National Resistance Movement, was probably given to him in his capacity as chairman of the local council, a position that suggested he was well-respected in the area. Augustino had a wife and seven children. Two of his grown daughters were staying in his home together with their ten children. It was a continuing struggle to support such a large household on his three acres of land; he had to rent fields from others, but managed to raise some crops for sale in order to cover school expenses for his many grandchildren. In the patrilineal Acholi society, the fathers of those children should have claimed them, even if they did not marry their mothers. But they did not even visit. As he said, 'I am like a slave working for children who belong elsewhere'. He had asked the fathers of the children – 'boys who loitered in the trading centre' – to take them; he had even spoken with their families, to no avail. Indeed, his daughters and his wife actively wanted to keep the children; they were not interested in filiating them to the fathers.

His suicide attempt a year earlier had failed and now, he assured us, he had resigned himself to live: 'If I am to die, let God take my life, not myself'. Things had erupted one evening when he went to the trading centre to visit his other wife. He had rented a room for her there because his first wife was unhappy about the liaison. On that evening she followed him angrily with a knife. In order to avoid a further spectacle, he returned home – his first wife behind him, quarrelling loudly. At home, his two grown daughters joined their mother, ganging up on him with words of abuse. Their betrayal – after all he had done for them and their children – angered him mightily. He rushed into the house and started to drink Ambush, the insecticide stored there, saying to his children, 'I am going to leave you to the happiness of the world'. He collapsed, spent two days in hospital, and recovered consciousness in time to sneak out before the police appeared to imprison him for the crime of attempting suicide.

Meanwhile, his wife ran away to her family in another district, fearing he would die and she would be blamed. When he finally went to bring her back, her family warned her against inciting violence and trying to stop her husband from doing what he wanted to do. But he has ended the relationship with the other woman, so that conflict has passed. He explained: 'A bitter heart (*cweer cwiny*) can have many sources ... You feel anger at yourself, anger at others and anger at the conditions. Anger (*kiniga*) can cause suicide. I have gotten over the anger, but what pains me most is my own children and wife turning against me'. Tears welled up in Augustino's eyes as he spoke.

Towards the end of our conversation, he looked behind us and saw his elder daughter going to harvest potatoes from the garden. 'She is bringing them to her lover in the trading centre. Yet she leaves her children here. She doesn't want to talk about it because it will bring quarrels.' Perhaps the situation galled him more sharply because his own biological father 'stole' in never marrying his mother or recognizing him as a son. He grew up in the home of his maternal grandfather. After his grandfather died, his mother's brothers turned against him and tried to force him off the land.

Augustino's tone when speaking of how his maternal uncles rejected him left no doubt about his bitterness. Now he was caring for his daughters' children as his own maternal grandfather had cared for him. The burden was onerous and he was unable to force the men who had 'stolen' his daughters to lift part of it. Even as an elected village council chairman he seemed incapable of exerting his authority – certainly not in the face of opposition by his wife and grown daughters. They humiliated him for taking a second woman, though this had always been the right of Acholi men. According to him, his wife's family had admonished her to maintain harmony by acquiescing to his wishes, but harmony of a sort was only re-established when he accepted her wishes.

It is noteworthy that Augustino's wife and daughters wanted to keep the children in their maternal home; they were not insisting that the biological fathers assume responsibility. Perhaps they did not judge the men capable of supporting the children. We see here the pattern of matrifocality that existed in the home of Noah, whose suicide we described at the outset of this chapter. The patrilineal virilocal configuration of gender relations, from which there had always been some divergences, is weakening. The shift has grave consequences for men who grow up in maternal homes where their claims to land are weak and where their very identity and belonging are questioned.

On another afternoon, a village counsellor brought us to Daniel at a trading centre where he repaired bicycles on the veranda of one of the shops. He moved deftly on crutches, one leg having been amputated below the knee, and he sat close to us since his hearing was poor after trying to kill himself with twelve tablets of quinine. Daniel told us how he had grown up with his mother's family. She died when he was a baby and his maternal grandmother cared for him. 'I was ten years old before I realized that I was in "a foreign land", that this was not my father's family.' Still, he got on well, he brought a wife, they built a house and a kitchen, and cultivated the land of his mother's brothers. He earned an income as a motorcycle taxi driver, which the entire family appreciated. Everything changed when he lost his leg after an accident. His wife left, his family turned their kitchen into a pig sty, things disappeared from his house. 'They loved me when I could contribute, but now I am a problem in my uncles' home.' Even his suicide failed. When he awoke with ringing ears after the overdose of quinine, he set his house alight in the hope of killing himself by fire. Everything burned except him. His mother's brothers took him to the police and wanted him imprisoned for suicide and arson, but the lay counsellor begged for his release. He could not rebuild his house because his missing leg left him unable to cut grass for thatch. He rented a room in the trading centre, but even that was a problem – he was no longer able to earn enough and could not keep up with the rent.

Daniel's unhappiness was compounded by several misfortunes: the loss of his leg and his wife's departure. But in telling his story, he put most weight on the problem of paternity, a gender problem that was not of his own making.

> They told me that I should look for my father but no one can tell me who my father is. Even my mother's mother says she doesn't know. Another problem is that my mother's mother married here when she already had my mother by another man. So my mother has a different father than my mother's brothers [they are half siblings, same mother different fathers]. It would be good if my father's family would pay compensation to my mother's family for bringing me up.

The lay counsellor, who was also a neighbour to Daniel, remarked: 'A child has a right to know his father, but some women hide the identity of the father because they are annoyed with him'.

In another paternity case, a village lay counsellor made the following entry into her notebook: 'Norbert wanted to kill himself because his father refused to pay his school fees and chased him away from his home while saying that N. was not his son. He should go and seek for his father elsewhere'. The predicaments of Daniel and Norbert were not simply economic; they were basically about not having a paternal family. Gender configurations do not only concern men's authority over their wives; they are also practices of generational filiation that pattern family identity and belonging.

While many homes struggled with scarce resources after the war and internment, we did not hear of men committing suicide because of poverty alone. Long ago, Paula Hirsch Foster put to Chief Jeremiah the question of whether poverty, the loss of all a man's property, would drive him to suicide. 'What about this, say your house burns down, and your fields do not bear and your cows all die, you become very very poor. Do you kill yourself for that?' He replied, 'No, that isn't enough to kill yourself for. If you are a strong man with no sickness you say: I can always get other wealth, and start working again. But in case your whole *gang* [home, family] dies in the fire, then that is enough for you to kill yourself too. You will say: Let me go together with my children, or with my brothers, whoever died'. In other words, it is family that sustains you, and losing them or being told that those you thought were family do not regard you as such is existentially a greater problem than poverty.

Figuring Configurations and Contaminations

Social scientists identify configurations as systems of institutions, norms, resources and relationships; indeed, finding patterns in social configurations of suicide has been their stock in trade since Émile Durkheim demonstrated how to study suicide as a social fact in 1897. There can be no doubt that the configuration of Acholi communal life and environment has been radically disturbed through the years of war. The title of Sverker Finnström's monograph (2008) on existence during the war years captures the reality of disorder and disaster: *Living with Bad Surroundings*. A configurational approach is holistic, reminding us that the contaminating effect of war plays out through an interconnected whole. Many aspects of social life are affected: political authority, livelihoods, resources, generational and gender relations. Researchers can 'objectively' characterize how these patterns of relationship are changing.

The extra work of ethnography in contrast to a more abstract assessment of systemic change is to show, as did Finnström, how our interlocutors figure it, how they problematize it, experience it and live with it. Construing configuration and contamination is an ongoing process undertaken by a variety of actors, not only academic analysts. Livingston's (2009) work on suicide in Botswana captures this very well, as she lays out different genres of suicide narratives told by and about middle-class Batswana. Although the situations she describes concerning consumption, personal indebtedness and investment in romantic relations gone awry differ from those in Acholiland, we appreciate her basic purpose to understand how Batswana construe: 'My aim ... is not so much to account for or to explain these suicides in sociological terms. Instead I am interested in how such suicides serve as a cautionary vehicle through which people contemplate and comment on what they see as the fundamental existential questions of their time...' (Livingston 2009: 659).

A recent monograph on suicide in Kerala takes a similar approach to figuring. Chua (2014) explicates professional and vernacular configurations of differential vulnerability to suicide. She shows how worries about exaggerated aspiration lead to the circulation of stereotypes about who are likely to kill themselves and why. People of lower castes and tribal people, who are used to life's harshness and do not have aspirations to 'middleclassness', are considered less vulnerable to suicide. Chua recognizes, however, that figuring suicide, making social interpretations in terms of over-ambition and unrealistic desires, reduces individual suffering to the categories and assumptions of common discourse. 'They push and mold individual cases of suicide to speak to and stand for ideas of social pathology and regional crisis ... [M]orality tales that locate the deaths of ... loved ones on the broad scales of social pathology flatten the complexities of individual and interpersonal suffering into generic scripts' (Chua 2014: 105).

There are levels and levels of figuring. Ugandan media reports have often interpreted the wave of suicides in the north as a consequence of the social disorder brought about by the war. Social scientists like Dolan, and clinical psychologists like Kizza and colleagues, figure northern Uganda suicide in terms of dislocations in gender roles and ideals. We too discern problematic and divergent expectations about gender relations that repeat as patterns across the cases we know. There would have been alternative ways of figuring. We considered changing patterns of alcohol consumption (Willis 2002) since heavy drinking played a role in so many suicides. Some of the newspaper reports pointed in that direction as well. Yet none of the individuals and families we talked to in depth mentioned alcohol as more than a facilitator of suicide, like the rope or the poison. Nor did families and individuals with whom we discussed personal experiences of suicide speak in general terms of the war or changing patterns of partnership and filiation of children. (The closest to such a generalization was uttered by Noah's mother who tried to halt his attack on his wife with the words: 'these days women are not quarrelled with like that'.)

Instead, they zoomed in on specific quarrels over resources and the paternity of certain children. They were concerned with very particular events, situations and circumstances, not generic patterns. In their telling, suicide was about relationships to intimate others and their responsibility for evoking bitterness and anger. Whereas the colonial and postcolonial governments made (attempted) suicide a crime committed by an individual, they considered the micro-configuration of family relations and the contaminating events as relevant to the allocation of blame. In our attempts to trace gender configurations, we wish to respect these complexities and the conjugations of each personal grief, while also trying to trace changing patterns of gender conflict and children's belonging.

Susan Reynolds Whyte
Professor, Department of Anthropology
University of Copenhagen, Denmark

Henry Oboke
Lecturer, Department of Mental Health
Lira University, Uganda

Notes

1. WHO (2019) figures show a similar increased frequency of male suicide globally, but with differences among countries. China, for example, has a more even sex distribution. While men predominate in 'successful' suicides, women more frequently attempt suicide, a phenomenon known as the 'gender paradox'.
2. Okumu had been a fighter in the LRA but he attributed his suicide attempt to the conflict with his wife rather than to the atrocities he experienced in the bush (Oboke and Whyte 2019).

References

Aber, Patience. 2012. 'Suicide on the Rise in Acholi Sub-region', *New Vision*, 22 October.

Akena, Moses, and Livingstone Kidega. 2012. 'Rising Suicide Cases Worry Gulu', *Daily Monitor*, 17 November.

Bohannon, Paul (ed.). [1960] 1967. *African Homicide and Suicide*. New York: Atheneum.

Bohannon, Paul. [1960] 1967. 'Patterns of Murder and Suicide', in Paul Bohannon (ed.), *African Homicide and Suicide*. New York: Atheneum, pp. 230–66.

Chua, Jocelyn Lim. 2014. *In Pursuit of the Good Life: Aspiration and Suicide in Globalizing South India*. Berkeley: University of California Press.

Connell, R.W., and James W. Messerschmidt. 2005. 'Hegemonic Masculinity: Rethinking the Concept', *Gender & Society* 19(6): 829–59.

Dolan, Chris. 2009. *Social Torture: The Case of Northern Uganda, 1986–2006*. New York: Berghahn Books.

Finnström, Sverker. 2008. *Living with Bad Surroundings: War, History and Everyday Moments in Northern Uganda*. Durham, NC: Duke University Press.

Girling, F.K. 1960. *The Acholi of Uganda*. London: Her Majesty's Stationery Office.

Kizza, Dorothy, et al. 2012a. 'Alcohol and Suicide in Postconflict Northern Uganda: A Qualitative Psychological Autopsy Study', *Crisis* 33: 95–105.

——— . 2012b. 'Men in Despair: A Qualitative Psychological Autopsy Study of Suicide in Northern Uganda', *Transcultural Psychiatry* 49(5): 696–717.

——— . 2012c. 'An Escape from Agony: A Qualitative Psychological Autopsy Study of Women's Suicide in a Post-conflict Northern Uganda', *International Journal of Qualitative Studies of Health and Well-Being* 7(18463). http//dx.doi.org/10.3402/qhw.v7i0.18463.

Lagace, Martha. 2014. 'A Historical Perspective on Gender Justice: How 1950s Acholi Women Advocated for Themselves with an Attitude of Calm Competence', *Voices* (7): 18–21.

Livingston, Julie. 2009. 'Suicide, Risk, and Investment in the Heart of the African Miracle', *Cultural Anthropology* 24(4): 652–80.

Niehaus, Isak. 2012. 'Gendered Endings: Narratives of Male and Female Suicides in the South African Lowveld', *Culture, Medicine and Psychiatry* 36(2): 327–47.

Obika, Julaina A., et al. 2018. 'Contesting Claims to Gardens and Land: Gendered Practice in Post-war Northern Uganda', in Patrick Cockburn et al. (eds), *Contested Property Claims: What Disagreement Tells Us about Ownership*. London: Routledge, pp. 205–20.

Oboke, Henry, and Susan R. Whyte. 2019. 'Anger and Bitter Hearts: The Spread of Suicide in Northern Ugandan Families', *Ethnos* 85(4): 612–28.

Owich, James. 2014. 'Nwoya Woman Survives Lynching after Husband Commits Suicide', *Acholi Times*, 10 November.

——— 2016. 'Nwoya Records over 60 Cases of Suicide', *Acholi Times*, 1 March.

Payne, Sarah, Viren Swami and Debbi L. Stanistreet. 2008. 'The Social Construction of Gender and Its Influence on Suicide: A Review of the Literature', *Journal of Men's Health* 5(1): 23–35.

Porter, Holly E. 2012. 'Justice and Rape on the Periphery: The Supremacy of Social Harmony in the Space between Local Solutions and Formal Judicial Systems in Northern Uganda', *Journal of Eastern African Studies* 6(1): 81–97.

——— 2016. *After Rape: Violence, Justice and Social Harmony in Northern Uganda*. Cambridge: Cambridge University Press.

Rosenberg, Charles E. 1992. *Explaining Epidemics and Other Studies in the History of Medicine*. Cambridge: Cambridge University Press.

Vaughan, Megan. 2010. 'Suicide in Late Colonial Africa: The Evidence of Inquests from Nyasaland', *American Historical Review* 115(2): 385–404.

Whyte, Susan Reynolds, et al. 2013. 'Remaining Internally Displaced: Missing Links to Human Security in Northern Uganda', *Journal of Refugee Studies* 26(2): 283–301.

Willis, Justin. 2002. *Potent Brews: A Social History of Alcohol in East Africa 1850–1999*. Oxford: James Currey.

World Health Organization. 2019. 'Mental Health. Suicide Crude Rates: Data Visualizations Dashboard, World Health Statistics 2019'. Retrieved 27 September 2019 from http://apps.who.int/gho/data/node.sdg.3-4-viz-2?lang=en.

Chapter 2
Configuring Epidemic Suicide in Oceania

Edward Lowe

In addition to its being an enduring human concern across time and space, suicide has been a central topic of study in the human sciences for over two centuries (Hacking 1990). The dominant understandings of suicide in the applied and theoretical social sciences can be found in psychology and psychiatry, on the one hand, and sociology, on the other. Given its status as the general science of the human condition, anthropology, surprisingly, has not had as much to say on the topic as these other fields (Staples and Widger 2012). However, this is beginning to change with several recent publications (e.g. Chua 2014; Staples and Widger 2012; Stevenson 2014; Widger 2015). I have also been writing about suicide and mental health for nearly two decades (Lowe 2003, 2019a, 2019b, 2020; Weisner and Lowe 2004). In this chapter, I aim to further the conversation regarding how an anthropology of suicide can offer a critically important perspective in relation to those already developed in other fields.

This chapter argues that both the ethnographic and comparative dimensions found in the emerging anthropology of suicide encourage a shift from a generalizing approach, where individual cases or societal statistics are 'read up' (Chua 2012) into pre-existing understandings of suicide as a phenomenon, to a configurational approach that emphasizes the diversity of suicidal phenomena as configurations of multiple factors that appear across social, cultural and historical contexts. Such an anthropological study of the diversities in global mental health is facilitated using the method of qualitative ethnographic comparison, which is often configurational in nature (Candea 2019; Gingrich 2012; Lowe and Schnegg 2020; Ragin 2014; Schnegg 2014; Seeberg and Meinert 2015). As Ragin (2014: x) notes, such a 'comparison allows the examination of constellations, configurations, and conjunctures. It is especially well suited for addressing questions about [how] different conditions combine in different and sometimes contradictory ways to produce the same or similar outcomes'.

To explore what a comparative and configurational approach in the anthropology of suicide might look like, the chapter uses the example of my own research on the suicide problem as it has emerged in the region of Oceania.[1] This project began in the mid to late 1990s when I conducted ethnographic research in Chuuk Lagoon on the social-relational dynamics that can lead to suicide as an endemic social practice. I chose Chuuk as a research site because it was one of the major Micronesian island groups where a well-documented suicide epidemic, sharply biased towards older teenage boys and young men, had been ongoing since the early 1970s. But unlike other Micronesian island groups, there is also a rich ethnographic literature from Chuuk Lagoon produced by psychological and medical anthropologists spanning a period of decades that allowed this case to be placed into a deeper ethnographic and historical context (e.g. Gladwin and Sarason 1953; Goodenough 1978; Hezel 1987; Marshall 1979; Rubinstein 1995).

The islands of Chuuk, and several other Micronesian islands, which were all part of the United Nations Trust Territory of the Pacific Islands that the United States administered from 1947 to 1987, were not the only islands in Oceania that had been experiencing a documented epidemic of suicide in the 1970s and 1980s. Samoa and Fiji were also sites of concern (Booth 1999; Bowles 1995; Haynes 1984; Macpherson and Macpherson 1987). The social scientific documentation of suicide on these islands followed publicly mediated accounts typically initiated by expatriate, American or Australian community-service workers, religious clergy and public health workers. The consensus view among these colonial and postcolonial agents was that rapid social changes associated with political independence, economic development and increasing globalization placed many indigenous people in Oceania at risk for a host of mental and physical health problems (e.g. Hezel

1976; Oliver 1985; Ward 2004). Eventually, publicly mediated accounts found in regional and global news outlets would frame extremely high rates of youth suicide as an outcome of either social disintegration or cultural disequilibrium that had resulted from late twentieth-century modernization and globalization (e.g. Field 2001; Wilson 2014).

One of the aims of this chapter is to place these universalizing accounts into proper context as components in a larger configurational framework that can be used to comparatively study suicide from anthropological and ethnographic standpoints. The sort of comparison I have in mind is a frontal type (Candea 2019) where the way a case is locally understood or configured is placed in explicit comparison with the assumptions that are dominant in the analyst's own lifeworld, in this case those that are dominant in academic research, international journalism, and the discourses of government ministries and international agencies. Human worlds are always foundationally intersubjective worlds. As a result, how we come to understand and explain epidemics is always interpenetrated by pre-existing, if often competing, discursive frames and heuristics. These competing frames of understanding do not exist on an even playing field, however. Powerful institutions and government agencies are interested in which discursive frameworks come to be dominant, as these often dovetail with governmental and international institutional agendas for (post)colonial governance (Miller and Rose 2008). We can study these framings in our ethnographic work by attending to publicly mediated accounts of modernization, globalization, and the potential harms they bring to local populations. Here, suicide is understood through an epidemic frame as a symptom of some alarming social condition that seems to have come about suddenly (Meinert and Seeberg, Introduction to this volume). Alternatively, these representations of suicide epidemics can articulate colonial and postcolonial anxieties about the ability of local, indigenous peoples to become independent modern societies in the western liberal style as opposed to recognizing the diverse modernities Oceanic peoples have already constructed for themselves (Hau'Ofa 1994; Lowe 2020). As such, the production of these publicly mediated discourses is part and parcel of enduring social and political inequalities in terms of who comes to be blamed for the problem.

A second aim of this chapter is to contrast the publicly mediated universalizing accounts of epidemic suicide with the way suicide is understood and configured within locally resonant understandings in Chuuk and elsewhere in Oceania. To do so, I explore ethnographically how suicide is understood as endemic in community and society through its local configuration within enduring forms of meaningful social practice and understanding (Malinowski [1926] 1949; Widger 2015). An important insight that emerges from attending to the configuration of local cases that are observed ethnographically is that suicides appear less an outcome of the sudden arrival of some sort of pathological societal condition but instead as an occasional 'presencing' (Heidegger 2000) that unfolds within diverse, ever unfolding and interlocking lifeworlds that made up the contexts of my fieldwork.

In the sections that follow, I bring these two aspects of the suicide problem in Chuuk and elsewhere in the region together to show how it came to be configured in this case and compare this configuration to ways it is often understood in (largely western) academic, therapeutic and other institutional contexts. First, I discuss the 'epidemic readings' (Chua 2012) of suicide in Oceania, where individual cases and epidemiological statistics for specific islands are 'read up' to fit them into universal explanations. Second, I present several cases showing how my local interlocutors in Chuuk and others in the region discuss suicide in endemic terms as occasional ruptures in what Oceanic people understand as a 'space of relating'. I will argue that the study of suicide in Oceania, and elsewhere, requires that we attend ethnographically and comparatively to the way suicide is configured discursively at different scales and how it is configured within everyday experience within local and regional lifeworlds.

Epidemic Readings of Suicide in Oceania

As Tom Widger (2015) has written, an ethnographic study of suicide and suicide epidemics shows that these are 'never a single event in time and space, but [are] rather deeply embedded in, and constitutive of on-going relationships across time and space – at the level of suicide events, lifespans, and history' (loc. 249). An anthropological study of suicide is something like stepping into an ongoing and unfolding stream of discourse and social production and trying to make some sense of the factors that give form to the patterns one documents over the course of time. My own ethnographic fieldwork on the suicide problem in Oceania began in 1995 with an initial trip to Chuuk Lagoon as a PhD student and continued actively through seven additional field stays over the course of the next twenty-two years. In those early years I imagined 'the field' as that part of my work that took place through interlocution and ethnographic encounters with people in the villages of Chuuk Lagoon where I mostly stayed. I have since come to think of ethnography not so much as 'being there' in a particular place that one designates as a field site, but in some sense 'stepping into' or 'living through' (Widger 2015) multiple streams of representation and practice that structured the problem of epidemic and endemic suicide in Chuuk and elsewhere. So, my own entry into the suicide problem in Chuuk in 1995 was to first step into a pre-existing network of academics, expatriate community workers, religious clergy and local elites who had already been engaged in an ongoing discussion of suicide in Micronesia and elsewhere in the Pacific for at least two and a half decades. Through these encounters, I came to understand the way in which the suicide epidemic was constructed metaphorically by members of this emergent network (Lowe 2020).

As an example of this network in action, consider how the anthropologist Martha Ward (2004) recounts an episode from her fieldwork on the Micronesian island of Pohnpei in 1970. She writes:

> the suicide rate particularly among young men had been climbing not just in Pohnpei but throughout Micronesia [in the late 1960s], there were reliable vital statistics and serious public health concerns, but no answers. Roger and I attended a funeral service for a teenager, the speakers attached the same complex causality to his suicide as they did for juvenile delinquency – modernization, breakdowns in traditions and in family life, pernicious Western influences, lack of community support systems, personal failings, and a decline of the work ethic. (79)

Between 1995 and 2008, I would encounter similar observations in my interlocutions among expatriates and locals living in various sites in Micronesia as we discussed news of the latest suicide death that reached us, whether these conversations took place on Pohnpei, in Chuuk Lagoon, on Guam, or on Majuro or Ebeye of the Marshall

Islands. These conversations had a familiar feel, often citing the same list of suspected causes that lay behind the suicide crisis that Ward recounts in her ethnographic memoir of that funeral on Pohnpei in 1970.

One can also find patterned and repetitive discourses in the mediated news reports that have appeared in the regional and international press over the decades. The earliest reports, with titles like 'Micronesia's Hanging Spree' (Hezel 1976) and 'Samoa's Youth Suicide Wave' (Va'a 1982) provide both individual cases and emerging epidemiological trends from island groups like Chuuk and Samoa, and then connect these to a narrative of 'modernization stress', either associated with notions of social disintegration or symbolic-regulatory (i.e. anomic) disequilibrium. More recently, reports have appeared in the news media with titles like 'Suicide the Way Out as Many Find Paradise Intolerable' (Field 2001) and 'Youth Suicides Sound Alarm across the Pacific' (Wilson 2014). While the earliest reports emplaced suicide on the islands where epidemiological trends had been documented, the empirical component of 'the suicide problem' in the more recent reporting is much murkier. As an example, in her 2014 report, Catherine Wilson leads her article with, 'Suicide rates in the Pacific Islands are some of the highest in the world and have reached up to 30 per 100,000 in countries such as Samoa, Guam and Micronesia, double the global average, with youth rates even higher'. Similarly, Michael Field (2001) reported to his international audience that, 'Samoans and Fiji Indians have the world's highest female suicide rates and the overall figures for the Federated States of Micronesia (FSM), the Marshall Islands, Samoa and Fiji are among the highest anywhere'. Neither Field (2001) nor Wilson informs their reader that the epidemiological studies that generated these statistics were from a period dating to the late 1970s to the early 1980s (Macpherson and Macpherson 1987; Rubinstein 1983), and after that time suicide rates declined on these islands substantially, particularly in Samoa (Booth 1999; Lowe 2019a).

These more recent reports also frame the reasons for the suicide problem in terms that are familiar to a western educated audience. For example, citing academic researchers in the region, Field (2001) diagnoses the suicide problem in ways that match well the discourse Martha Ward (2004) reported from her fieldwork three decades earlier. Field (2001) quotes an academic who claimed, 'A major cause has been diagnosed as the erosion of social structures and values, leaving many young people marginalized and insecure'. While Field takes up the argument from the standpoint of social and cultural disintegration, Catherine Wilson adopts the 'failed development' and increased anomie or symbolic-regulatory disequilibrium discourse. She writes, 'The United Nations Children's Fund (UNICEF) warns that "denial of economic and social opportunities leads to frustrated young people" and "the result can be a high incidence of self-harm" with "the loss of the productive potential of a large section of the adult population"' (Wilson 2014). Earlier, Wilson suggests that while rapid globalization generates 'new aspirations' among young people, the lack of means to realize these new aspirations leads to frustration, psychosocial distress and increased vulnerability to suicide.

In the 1980s and 1990s, these enduring discursive frames had also circulated through the academic scholarship concerning suicide in the region (Booth 1999; Haynes 1984; Hezel 1987; Macpherson and Macpherson 1987; Rubinstein 1983). It is likely that these academic sources then informed the sources relied upon by journalists like Field and Wilson. Earlier publicly mediated accounts that had appeared in regional news publications in the late 1970s and early 1980s likely also influenced later reporting. Looking back at these earlier news articles (Hezel 1976; Va'a 1982), one finds the same explanatory discourses that would appear in reporting later.

This phase of my own anthropology of the suicide problem in Oceania fits well with the approach taken by Jocelyn Chua (2012) in her study of the suicide and aspirational culture she encountered in Kerala, India. In that work, Chua describes 'epidemic readings' of suicide cases. Staples and Widger (2012) summarize Chua's argument as follows:

> Bodies dead from suicide are not ... interpreted and mourned solely in terms of their own histories, but are read 'up' to fit, and to stand in for, aggregate trends: what she terms 'epidemic readings' of suicide. The death of, say, a student, might be categorised in ways that speak to wider issues concerning pressure on young people to achieve academically, to the problem of failed love affairs, to changed financial circumstances, and, more generally, to overriding themes – discussed ad nauseam in the South Indian media – of social decline. (Staples and Widger 2012: 190–91)

But in the case of publicly mediated discourses of the suicide problem in Oceania, it is not only individual cases that are read up to fit into broader categories and theories that explain suicide in universal terms, but epidemic rates of suicide for entire countries or regions can be read this way. These discourses tend to emphasize both social decline and failed modernization as explanatory tropes, typically blaming indigenous leaders or parents for both decline and failure to properly develop into modern westernized liberal societies (Lowe 2020). They therefore serve the dominant political and economic interests of regional powers like France, the United States, Australia, New Zealand and the United Kingdom. These are the very powers that controlled the various island groups just prior to the period of political indigenization from the 1950s to the 1980s.

Endemic Suicide in the Space of Relating

Beyond the encounters with institutional and publicly mediated discourses of suicide, when studying a suicide problem ethnographically one also inevitably encounters cases where someone has died of a suicide attempt in their field site (Chua 2014; Widger 2015). These events, while tragic, provide an opportunity to shift from encounters with globalizing discourses and the associated epistemologies of powerfully positioned institutional actors to epistemologies and configurations of lived experience that reflect local and regional lifeworlds, epistemologies that are more experience-near to suicide as a phenomenon rather than a metaphor for societal disturbance in the face of late twentieth-century neoliberal modernization programmes. While it is rare to directly witness the occasions that could lead to potentially lethal deliberate acts of self-harm, one does regularly encounter forms of everyday talk and ritual practice around cases that have occurred recently. Such ethnographic encounters allow one to see, as Tom Widger (2015) has noted, how people live through suicides as historical events and as a more general community problem. The ethnographic encounter with suicide *in situ* allows one to investigate the ways in which it is configured within social, cultural and historical contexts that are generally not available to either clinical or survey researchers.

When encountering cases of suicide and the way these cases were narrated and problematized through everyday conversation by people in the villages where I and other researchers conducted fieldwork in Chuuk and elsewhere in the region, I was always struck by how they contrasted with accounts that were familiar to me in the United States, where suicide cases are often narrated in highly individualized ways. Suicides are said to be occasioned by such things as 'romantic failures or upheavals, economic and job setbacks, confrontations with the law, terminal or debilitating illnesses, situations that cause great shame ... the injudicious use of alcohol or drugs' (Redfield-Jamison 1999: 19).

The motive for suicide is often understood by suicidologists in the United States to be related to a person trying to cope with intense intrapsychic pain. The suicidologist Edwin Schneidman (1996) labelled the sort of psychic pain that is often thought to accompany suicide as 'psychache', which he described as intense psychic pain that can entirely consume the mind. This pain is intrinsic to psychological processes, often reflecting excessive feelings of shame, guilt, fear, anxiety, loneliness or dread. Its introspective nature is undeniable, Schneidman continues; suicide can occur when this psychache becomes so unbearable that death is actively sought to end the unceasingly painful consciousness. He concludes that '*suicide is the tragic drama in the mind*' (13, emphasis added).

These ways of understanding suicide are consonant with some well-known sociological definitions of the modern self (Giddens 1991; Taylor 1989). Suicide for many in the west is understood as an ending of one's biography, particularly one characterized by intense and enduring psychological pain. As one colleague commented in reference to an earlier presentation of this chapter, suicide is understood in the west as 'the obliteration of the self' through an intentional act of lethal self-harm.

These characterizations by American specialists do not fit well with the understanding afforded me through ethnographic encounters I have recorded from Chuuk and those that others report both for Chuuk and in places like Samoa and elsewhere in the region (Hollan 1990; Macpherson and Macpherson 1987). Instead, in many Oceanic and Austronesian communities, suicide attempts are typically understood to have emerged at the nexus of acute disruptions in the reciprocal flows of social relatedness that almost always involve close kin. Indeed, in Chuuk, suicide is understood as just one outcome of a more general practice for negotiating crises in relationships that occasionally erupt among close kin. This more general practice is called *amwuunamwuun* in Chuuk. Rubinstein (1995: 32) describes *amwuunamwuun* as refusing 'to talk to others, to isolate themselves and avoid contact with others, perhaps to refuse to eat, and as an ultimate expression of their emotional state, to [attempt to] kill themselves'. The main aim here is to make an appeal to the offending person or to some other kin who can help with the conflict to mend the damaged relationship. This may be achieved by removing oneself from the scene so the offending other might feel shame or regret over the conflict. Rubinstein (1995) notes further that this situation could, ideally, end happily with reconciliation, often with another relative who might chase after the fleeing person, and using soft words and kindness bring them back to the family where apologies and nurturing care might resume. But all too often it ends with potentially lethal acts of self-harm, particularly in the case of older teens and young adults.

We can see these social-relational dynamics in several cases that are reported from Chuuk. Consider the following three cases as typical examples.

Case 1

On 19 June 1996, I wrote about the following case in my fieldnotes. The case involved the fifteen-year-old second son of one of the men in my host's matrilineage. According to several interlocutors, the story of the death went something like the following: while working to make breadfruit pudding (a local staple) for the family last Saturday, the boy and his work companion got into a fight. Somehow his mother got involved and slapped her son. The boy was angry, possibly ashamed, and went off into the bush. There, he found some rope, took off his shirt and hanged himself. In discussing this case, an older teenage boy told me that the victim's work companion saw his mother slap him and that this may have had something to do with the case as such an event can cause acute shame or embarrassment. Many described the victim as a nice and funny boy, but when he was angry he could be a little crazy or uncontrolled (*umwes*). Talking about the case with another teen and a young man from the victim's larger kin group in the evening, there seemed to be some opinion that the victim was just going to attempt suicide but did not intend to die. But once he leaned into the rope he lost consciousness and died. The two seemed to share an understanding that this style of hanging is painless, and one dies because she or he loses consciousness and is 'at peace' (*kinamue*). Therefore, they cannot change their minds before they lose consciousness.

Case 2

The anthropologist Don Rubinstein (1995: 28–29) reported the case of an older teen named Sima who lived on the island of Uman in Chuuk Lagoon and who committed suicide in 1990. In this case, the trouble began during a time when Sima and his family had left his mother's village to join the entire family in his father's family village for the funeral of Sima's paternal grandmother. Sima was unhappy with the sudden change in arrangements and felt uncomfortable among so many of his father's relatives. Sima's father was keen to demonstrate his filial responsibilities to his mother's kin. So, he became quite demanding, requiring Sima to work long hours hauling coral boulders to build a seawall around his father's older brother's house. Sima was seen venting his unhappiness on a few occasions by uncharacteristically shouting insults at people along the path. Sima's suicide took place on a Saturday morning. The night before, Sima's father had ordered Sima to wake early to help prepare breadfruit pudding (*kkón*), so that the family was well fed on Sunday, a day of rest in Chuuk. That morning, Sima's father asked him and a friend to go into the village to borrow the long bamboo hooked pole that is used to harvest breadfruit. But the two youths dawdled while in the village and eventually returned empty handed. Sima's father was furious and scolded Sima severely. He even waved his machete in Sima's face, threatening to chase his son with the knife before irately telling the boy to 'Get out of here, and go find somewhere else to live!' (Rubinstein 1995: 28). Rubinstein reports that Sima and his friend withdrew, with Sima telling the other youth to return to his home alone. Sima travelled tearfully back to his own house in his mother's village, which had been temporarily vacated during the funeral period. He encountered his younger brother along the path and borrowed a pen. A few hours later, the younger brother went looking for Sima. As he was not seen along the village path, the boy guessed that Sima might be back in their house in their own village. Looking inside, he saw the figure of Sima in a dark room, apparently standing, but with an odd, slack posture. He found a way into the house and started screaming when he realized that Sima had hanged himself.

Case 3
Both the case that I recorded in 1996 and the one Rubinstein recorded in 1990 took place during the suicide epidemic that had been ongoing since the early 1970s. Thomas Gladwin (Gladwin and Sarason 1953: 145–46) also recorded a case of *amwuunamwuun* that he witnessed during his ethnographic fieldwork in Chuuk Lagoon nearly fifty years earlier during his fieldwork in the period just after the Second World War, well before the onset of the suicide epidemic in Chuuk. The case involved a young man named Andy and the trouble started when he argued with his mother over the repair of a pillow. The argument became heated and Andy's father's sister, who was also present during the argument, accused Andy of being a bad son. After that accusation, Andy left the house with what Gladwin described as a look of almost hysterical desperation on his face. Andy picked up a large stick and used it to beat on the side of the house several times. He then dropped the stick and quickly climbed to the top of a tall coconut tree. Andy was followed by a relative who pleaded with the youth to come to his senses. Andy paused for a moment but then swung out onto a frond of the tree, threatening to jump. Gladwin jumped to action, placing himself under the tree to prevent the youth from jumping. Andy stayed in the tree for about twenty minutes more, sobbing openly before being persuaded to come down by another older relative.

How are we to make sense of these three cases? Both the psychological and sociological perspectives take as their point of departure an epidemic reading of suicide, where these cases of suicide might be understood as indicative of a more general reaction to or consequence of an apparent increase in pathological, sociological, psychological and pathophysiological conditions in these communities. But an anthropological sensitivity to the way local people in Oceania understand the cases presented above points instead to a durable social-relational practice that is present in places like Chuuk before and after the emergence of the empirically documented suicide epidemic of the last decades of the twentieth century. This ethnographic reading suggests the possibility of an *endemic* relational social practice that is locally enduring if also historically contingent in terms of its intensity (Malinowski [1926] 1949; Widger 2015). As noted earlier, in Chuuk this practice is called *amwuunamwuun* and only occasionally results in lethal acts of self-harm.

The idea that suicide can be a form of social practice has its origins in an analysis of a suicide case that Bronislaw Malinowski ([1926] 1949) documented in his fieldwork on the Trobriand islands in the early twentieth century. Staples and Widger (2012: 192) summarize Malinowski's argument as follows:

> Acts of suicidal behaviour, when performed under certain conditions and when employing certain kinds of methods, are well known to act as a kind of complaint or challenge to specific others, with whom the suicidal individual is in some quarrel. By attempting or committing suicide, the individual lays blame upon those others, who by social convention the kinsmen of the suicidal person are now compelled to seek revenge upon. Thus, not only is the suicidal person absolved of his or her crime, but culpability for it, in one way or another, passes to other people.

Other ethnographic studies of suicide would confirm Malinowski's argument as far as seeing suicide as a recognized means of protesting some perceived injustice or insult. In many places around the world, suicide is 'a socially legitimate means of protest when other, more "direct" forms are not allowed by social convention, for example in the context of gender inequality' (Staples and Widger 2012: 192). But local understandings of *amwuunamwuun* practice and the potentially lethal acts of self-harm that can accompany these episodes are not understood in Chuuk or elsewhere in Oceania as acts of 'revenge' (Gerber 1985; Rubinstein 1995). As I will show below, these acts are often desperate attempts to restore reciprocal relational flows among close kin of care, respect and support that have suddenly broken down.

I should emphasize here that my argument is not that suicide and self-harm can never be an indication of psychological, psychiatric or sociological pathology. Rather, as Staples and Widger (2012) argue, the anthropology of suicide goes beyond these explanations to suggest that in many contexts suicidal behaviour is a form of social practice that speaks to conditions of inequality and injustice, particularly when other means of airing grievances are limited. To view suicide in strictly pathological terms is to both deny the victim agency and direct attention away from the political-economic dimensions of suicide and other acts of self-harm.

Self-Harm and the Dynamics of the Space-of-Relating in Oceania

Comparing the material from Chuuk to other examples given in the recent literature from Oceania, we can see that suicide in the region is not configured in terms of the reflexive, inward-focused biographical self that one intentionally 'obliterates' in a final act of self-definition given a state of intolerable psychological pain. Indeed, given the widespread understanding in Chuuk and elsewhere in the region that one continues to have an active, intentional role in the affairs of living kin as either a 'good' or 'bad' spirit after death (Goodenough 2002; Lowe 2018), there is no sense that one's self can possibly be 'obliterated'. Such a notion is a culture-bound invention of the west dating back at least to the eighth-century BCE Greeks (Arendt 1958; cf. Geertz 1983; Strathern 1988).

Instead, we can view general practices like *amwuunamwuun* and more specific, lethal practices of self-harm from a more locally resonant epistemological standpoint as reflecting a rupture in what many indigenous Oceanic scholars have recently called 'the space of relating'. This concept refers to an understanding of social being-in-the-world that is quite widespread in Oceania and that continues to inform expressions of Oceanic modernity (e.g. HauʻOfa 1994; Lilomaiava-Doktor 2009; Mila-Schaaf 2006). Thus, a reading of suicide that draws on the recent scholarship of indigenous Oceanic scholars themselves and developments in phenomenological anthropology (e.g. Zigon 2007) would frame suicide as a social practice that emerges during a sudden breakdown in the space of relating.

Karlo Mila (Mila-Schaaf 2006) reviews the relatively recent literature on the space of relating and its importance for accurately describing experiences of self and identity that are widespread among Oceanic societies. In many of these communities, self is understood as emerging not from a reflexive sense of one's own biography, but within a space of relating to others in one's phenomenal world. In the space of relating, self is typically forged in 'relationship, interaction, interconnection, and belonging' (Mila-Schaaf 2006: 11). An important dimension of the space of relating in Oceanic communities is that it must be constantly created and maintained. Like the boundaries of gardens between neighbours, Mila-Schaaf (2006) notes, maintaining the space of relating 'requires [constant] effort. It means that one ensures that one's relationships with others are sound. One meets obligations. One respects the other and ensures balanced reciprocity of giving and taking' (11).

The space of relating then is accompanied by a general aesthetic of balanced reciprocity, even in hierarchical relationships. This aesthetic informs 'a code of ideal and expected behaviour between people, between brothers and sisters, fathers and daughters, aunts and nieces, community to community, stranger to stranger. [This] is the space between people, the dynamic of relationship, that is what happens between you and me' (Mila-Schaaf 2006: 10–11). The sort of reciprocal flows of care and respect that create and sustain a harmonious space of relating and that fundamentally inform notions of moral personhood among those who are enmeshed in its practices is foundational to the production of a sense of moral being-in-the-world in places like Chuuk and elsewhere.

This sense of nurturing relationships as a means of fashioning morally resonant spaces of relating was made clear to me often in formal interviews with people in Chuuk about the relational dynamics that might lead to suicide. Before discussing suicide, I began our conversations by asking about the key moral term in Chuuk, *ttong* (compassion, love), which is used in everyday life to describe the ideal state for all positive human relationships. The way *ttong* is ideally produced through acts of support and care among kin and non-kin alike in Chuuk was made clear in the following response by Kimura, a 67-year-old man, when responding to my question, 'How does a man show *ttong* to his family?' Here is how Kimura responded:

> Kimura: A father can show his love for his children, in the tradition of the old days, those things that are important, his children will have.
> I: Like what? What kinds of things?
> Kimura: Land, that is the most important thing above all. Because that is the life of the people of Chuuk. ... On account of land, I will feed my children ... what my child values, I will give them. Whatever the son wants, I will get. If he has brothers or a sister, I will say ... you will take care of your sisters there first and share together. You ... will see what

their needs are. Regarding women, she will take hold of those things that reflect the responsibility of a woman ... out on the reef. The woman will take care, will go and fish. She will tell her younger sisters, you will feed your brothers, your fathers, the matrilineal relatives. If she has sisters, she will feed her sisters.

I: This is concerning the work on the ocean, but what about the responsibilities of men?

Kimura: I am also able to tell him, you will pound breadfruit and make the earth oven (*wuum*). You will feed your fathers, your brothers. You will feed your sisters, your mothers. If they also have children, they will feed them. That is how they have peace (*kinamue*) together. But he will just look toward his fathers, will just look after them. He will just work hard, take care of them. Because, if he does not take care of the *samon* (lineage chief), then there will not be anyone who will want to help him. There will not be someone who feels *ttong* for him. But, if there is just helpfulness [*aninisééch*], everyone will feel *ttong* for him. That is the reason that in tradition everyone will just work hard, because there will be hope [*epinukunuk*] that there will be someone's love for him/her.

Here, Kimura frames his response in terms of the importance of nurturing a wide set of relationships through hard work and service to others in one's kin group on an ongoing basis. Through reciprocal acts of care and work, one builds peace (*kinamue*) in the space of relating and can also be optimistic (*epinukunuk*) that others care for her or him. Elsewhere in the interviews we discussed episodes where such faith in the caring and compassion of others in one's networks of belonging breaks down, where efforts made are not adequately reciprocated and the trouble (*osukosuk*) and hurt feelings that can then emerge because of such conditions of some disturbance in the reciprocal flows of relating. It was in the context of such moments of breakdown that Kimura would go on to describe episodes of *amwuunamwuun*.

Suicide Practice That Results from Moments of Moral Breakdown

Looking back at each of the cases of suicide described earlier, we can interpret them as arising out of sudden ruptures in the flows that would characterize more harmonious spaces of relating. In a sense, these moments follow from moments of moral breakdown, a term the anthropologist Jarrett Zigon (2007) developed from his reading of the philosophers Husserl, Heidegger and Dreyfus. Zigon describes his concept of the moral breakdown in typically western terms, as a dynamic that is internal to the individual. He writes:

> my research ... suggests that most people consider others and themselves moral most of the time, and for this reason it is rarely considered or consciously thought about ... The need to consciously consider or reason about what one must do only arises in moments that shake one out of the everydayness of being moral. This moment is what I will call ... the moral breakdown. (2007: 133)

In the context of the way local people in Chuuk and elsewhere in Oceania talk about suicide, a sense of moral personhood is not understood as an internal psychological state of the individual. Rather it is understood dynamically and relationally through an ongoing production of relatedness through flows of interchange in one's networks of belonging. The situations described in each of the suicide cases given above are indeed moments of moral breakdown, not exclusively in the experience of the suicide victim, but in the entire space of relating that is active during the event that immediately precedes the attempted act of self-harm.

With this reading in mind, we might see the act of self-harm in places like Chuuk *not* as an attempt to get relief from intense intrapsychic pain, but more in the sense of what Edward Hagen and colleagues (2008) have called 'costly signalling'. Acts of deliberate self-harm in this context send a credible signal to the members of one's space of relating that disturbances in harmonious reciprocal flows that are an ideal state for the space of relating threaten the well-being of its members, particularly those who occupy subaltern positions such as older teens and young adults relative to their older siblings or parents. Such credible signals to others may have the aim of motivating others to intervene and mend the imbalance or rupture that has suddenly broken out into the open in the relationship. We see in the case of Andy reported by Tom Gladwin just this sort of intervention enacted. Andy's relatives chased after him to try and get him to pause as he climbed to the top of a coconut tree with the intention of throwing himself from its crown. Later, another relative was able to eventually convince Andy to come down. If Andy's case is anything like the dozens of family conflicts in Chuuk that I have witnessed, Andy will be expected to apologize to his family and they in turn will apologize to him. But even in cases where an act of deliberate self-harm proves lethal, the kin group of the victim will meet the evening before the funeral and burial to air any grievances that they have with each other and apologize, thereby restoring a sense of love and respect among the kin network that has assembled for the funeral (Lowe 2018). Such moments of 'disentangling relations' [*tafa ewe nefin*], as it is called in Chuuk, not only aim to restore harmonious reciprocal relating among living kin, but also in the relation of living kin to the spirits of deceased kin, including the victims of suicide.

Conclusion

In this chapter I present two elements of a general framework that can be used to study suicide epidemics anthropologically.[2] The first element explored how suicide cases can be incorporated into epidemic readings of suicide that are often found in publicly mediated accounts, whether these are found in academic publications, the institutional grey literature, or regional or global news outlets. Here, individual cases are read up in order to fit them into pre-existing dominant theories of suicide as a universal phenomenon. The universal theories emphasized in these accounts often favour the policy agendas and politics of powerful governmental and non-governmental agents and institutions that connect suicide to social decline and failed modernization. Too often the blame is placed on indigenous people for the situation, while eliding the responsibility of various postcolonial or neocolonial agents (Lowe 2020).

The second element explored how suicide as an endemic condition is locally configured through enduring forms of meaningful social practice and understanding (Malinowski [1926] 1949; Widger 2015). This endemic reading shows that suicides appear less an outcome of the sudden arrival of some sort of pathological societal condition but instead more like what Heidegger (2000) called the 'presencing' of phenomena, by which he meant that appearances (like cases of suicide) are presences of larger, less immediately apparent processes of human being-in-the-world. In this chapter, I showed how the appearance of suicide is a potentiality present in the endemic social practice of *amwuunamwuun* in Chuuk.

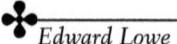
Edward Lowe

Amwuunamwuun practice is, in turn, an emergent potentiality that is found in moments of moral breakdown in the social-relational flows that constitute the construction of spaces of relating in these islands. Suicide in Chuuk can become a presence in social life as part of the attempt to restore harmony in the space of relating after a disturbance. This contrasts with the understanding of suicide dominant in the United States, where suicide is seen as a potentiality that arises from seeking relief from intense intrapsychic pain that can occur due to a breakdown in everyday acts of self-making that make up the fashioning of an individual's lived biography, an understanding that is often found in the publicly mediated accounts of suicide in Oceania given by western writers.

Overall, then, we might view suicide both as a discursive metaphor and as a phenomenon in lived experience as presences that unfold within the diverse and interlocking lifeworlds that one can and does encounter through ethnographic fieldwork. The key to their analysis and interpretation is to try and understand through comparative ethnographic analysis the way those lifeworlds come to be configured such that a phenomenon like suicide can appear as metaphorical/discursive, endemic behavioural, and epidemic phenomena, but that these become presences through different processes depending on the context and scale of the phenomena.

So, what does the preceding say about the main themes for this volume of configuration and contagion? I have provided a configurational account of endemic and epidemic suicide in Oceania that suggests that conditions can combine in different ways across contexts to produce seemingly similar epidemic outcomes. The upshot of this is that we must attend closely to contexts of configuration if we are to understand better biosocial and psychosocial epidemics. We must also do so comparatively, critically and reflexively because, as noted earlier, human worlds are always foundationally intersubjective worlds, with the corollary implication that the ways people come to understand and explain epidemics are always interpenetrated by pre-existing, if often competing, discursive frames and heuristics. Powerful international and post- or neocolonial institutions have an interest in which discursive frameworks are adopted, creating powerful incentives to adopt universalizing epistemological and explanatory frameworks that are often used within these institutional networks. In contrast, I have attempted here to show the way in which I have attended to the suicide epidemic in Chuuk as it 'presences' (Heidegger 2000) discursively and phenomenologically within the diverse, ever unfolding and interlocking lifeworlds that made up the contexts of my fieldwork.

Finally, reflecting on Heidegger's notion that appearances in the world as phenomena are presences of larger processes of being, I find that this chapter provides a useful empirical example for exploring the productive tensions and conjunctions between concepts of contagion and configuration in the study of biosocial epidemics that Meinert and Seeberg usefully describe in the Introduction to this volume. From a phenomenological perspective, I wonder if epidemic rates of biosocial and psychosocial disease or problems like suicide can be seen to reflect the spread through populations (as if they were little units that are transported from one body to another) as opposed to intensified presences within them. If we are not careful in our understanding of contagion, we might privilege a reductive biomechanical ontology and scientific epistemology that is so often the handmaiden of various forms of modern colonialism past and present (Miller and Rose 2008). As I suggest here, and as Meinert and Seeberg also suggest in their Introduction, perhaps it is better to think of disease epidemics as an *intensification* of locally configured presences of illness-related phenomena in the hierarchically interpenetrated configured conditions of human lifeworlds. If this is the case, then we should adopt methods that encourage us to attend carefully in a sustained fashion to the way biosocial and psychosocial epidemics appear within human lifeworlds such that we can better apprehend the underlying processes that configure their appearances.

Acknowledgements

I would like to thank three anonymous reviewers, Jens Seeberg, Lotte Meinert, Cheryl Mattingly, Andrea Chiovenda, Byron Good, Mary-Jo del Vecchio-Good and Michael M.J. Fischer for their very helpful comments on earlier drafts of this manuscript. I am also grateful for the many years of support and continuing education provided to me by many people who live on the islands of Chuuk Lagoon. Mr Amanisio Joseph and Mr Benisio Joseph have been particularly helpful over the years, as well as members of their families and wider kin groups. Portions of this research were funded by the Wenner-Gren Foundation (Grant No. 6126), the National Science Foundation (SBR-9529185), and the Pacific Basin Research Center (2012 Summer Grant).

Edward Lowe
Professor of Anthropology
Soka University of America, USA

Notes

1. In this chapter, I adopt Epeli Hau'Ofa's (1994) labelling of the region that includes the Pacific Islands settled by Papuan and Oceanic speakers as *Oceania* rather than the more traditional western label of the *Pacific Islands*. The former emphasizes regional mobilities and interconnections, which have always characterized the lives of Oceanic people. The latter imports a western trope of isolation, immobility and backwardness.
2. A third element of this framework, which I discuss elsewhere (Lowe 2019a, 2019b), is to consider the larger scalar processes and world unfolding that can lead to an increased intensity of endemic suicide such that it produces a sudden increase in the suicide rate (i.e. an epidemic of suicide). In this work, I show that dominant universal explanations do not fit the empirical patterns for epidemics in places like Samoa and in the island polities of Micronesia. Instead, different factors associated with diverse local responses, processes of globalization and neoliberalization of the global economy and its political-economic structures matter more.

References

Arendt, Hannah. 1958. *The Human Condition*. Chicago: University of Chicago Press.

Booth, Heather. 1999. 'Pacific Island Suicide in Comparative Perspective', *Journal of Biosocial Science* 31(4): 433–48.

Bowles, John. 1995. 'Suicide in Western Samoa: An Example of a Suicide Prevention Programme in a Developing Country', in R. Diekstra et al. (eds), *Preventative Strategies on Suicide*. Leiden, NL: Brill Academic Publishers, pp. 173–206.

Candea, Matei. 2019. *Comparison in Anthropology: The Impossible Method*. Cambridge: Cambridge University Press.

Chua, Jocelyn Lim. 2012. 'Tales of Decline: Reading Social Pathology into Individual Suicide in South India', *Culture, Medicine, and Psychiatry* 36(2): 204–24.

———. 2014. *In Pursuit of the Good Life: Aspiration and Suicide in Globalizing South India*. Berkeley: University of California Press.

Durkheim, Emile. 1951. *Suicide: A Study in Sociology*, trans. J.A. Spaulding. New York: The Free Press.

Field, Michael. 2001. 'Suicide the Way Out as Many Find Paradise Intolerable'. Agence France Presse, 12 November. Retrieved 6 July 2016 from Google database.

Geertz, Clifford. 1983. *Local Knowledge: Further Essays in Interpretive Anthropology*. New York: Basic Books.

Gerber, Elinor R. 1985. 'Rage and Obligation: Samoan Emotion in Conflict', in G.M. White and J. Kirkpatrick (eds), *Person, Self, and Experience: Exploring Pacific Ethnopsychologies*. Berkeley: University of California Press, pp. 121–167.

Giddens, Anthony. 1991. *Modernity and Self-Identity: Self and Society in the Late Modern Age*. Cambridge: Polity Press.

Gingrich, Andre. 2012. 'Comparative Methods in Socio-Cultural Anthropology Today', in R. Fardon et al. (eds), *The SAGE Handbook of Social Anthropology*. Los Angeles: Sage, pp. 211–22.

Gladwin, Thomas, and Seymour B. Sarason. 1953. *Truk: Man in Paradise*. Viking Fund Publications 20. New York: Wenner-Gren Foundation for Anthropological Research, Inc.

Goodenough, Ward H. 1978. *Property, Kin, and Community on Truk*, 2nd edn. New York: Archón Books.

———. 2002. *Under Heaven's Brow: Pre-Christian Religious Tradition in Chuuk*. Philadelphia: American Philosophical Society.

Hacking, Ian. 1990. *The Taming of Chance*. Cambridge: Cambridge University Press.

Hagen, Edward H., Paul J. Watson and Peter Hammerstein. 2008. 'Gestures of Despair and Hope: A View on Deliberate Self-Harm from Economics and Evolutionary Biology', *Biological Theory* 3(2): 123–38.

Hau'ofa, Epeli. 1994. 'Our Sea of Islands', *The Contemporary Pacific* 6(1): 148–61.

Haynes, Ruth H. 1984. 'Suicide in Fiji: A Preliminary Study', *British Journal of Psychiatry* 145(4): 433–38.

Heidegger, Martin. 2000. *Introduction to Metaphysics*. New Haven, CT: Yale University Press.

Hezel, Francis X. 1976. 'Micronesia's Hanging Spree'. *Micronesian Independent*, 31 December. Retrieved 6 July 2016 from Google database.

———. 1987. 'Truk Suicide Epidemic and Social Change', *Human Organization* 46(4): 283–91.

Hollan, Douglas. 1990. 'Indignant Suicide in the Pacific: An Example from the Toraja Highlands of Indonesia', *Culture, Medicine and Psychiatry* 14(3): 365–79.

Lilomaiava-Doktor, Sa'iliemanu. 2009. 'Beyond "Migration": Samoan Population Movement (Malaga) and the Geography of Social Space (Vā)', *The Contemporary Pacific* 21(1): 1–32.

Lowe, Edward D. 2003. 'Identity, Activity, and the Well-Being of Adolescents and Youth: Lessons from Young People in a Micronesian Society', *Culture Medicine and Psychiatry* 27(2): 187–219.

———. 2018. 'Kinship, Funerals and the Durability of Culture in Chuuk', in N. Quinn (ed.), *Advances in Culture Theory from Psychological Anthropology*. Mind and Society Series. Palgrave MacMillan, pp. 75–107.

———. 2019a. 'Epidemic Suicide in the Context of Modernizing Social Change in Oceania: A Critical Review and Assessment', *The Contemporary Pacific* 31(1): 105–38.

———. 2019b. 'Social Change and Micronesian Suicide Mortality: A Test of Competing Hypotheses', *Cross-Cultural Research* 53(1): 3–32.

———. 2020. 'Suicide Epidemics, Post-Colonial Governance, and the Image of the Recalcitrant Native in Oceania', in A. Patterson and I. Read (eds), *The SHAPES of Epidemics and Global Disease*. Newcastle upon Tyne: Cambridge Scholars Publishing, pp. 64–86.

Lowe, Edward D., and Michael Schnegg. 2020. 'Comparative Ethnography: Its Promise, Process, and Successful Implementations', in M. Schnegg and E.D. Lowe (eds), *Comparing Cultures: Innovations in Comparative Ethnography*. Cambridge: Cambridge University Press, pp. 1–20.

Macpherson, Cluny, and La'avasa Macpherson. 1987. 'Towards an Explanation of Recent Trends in Suicide in Western Samoa', *Man* 22(2): 305–30.

Malinowski, Bronislaw. [1926] 1949. *Crime and Custom in Savage Society*. London: Routledge & Kegan Paul.

Marshall, Mac. 1979. *Weekend Warriors: Alcohol in a Micronesian Culture*. Palo Alto, CA: Mayfield Publishing Company.

Mila-Schaaf, Karlo. 2006. 'Vā-Centered Social Work: Possibilities for a Pacific Approach to Social Work Practice', *Social Work Review* (Ti Mau II) 18(1): 8–13.

Miller, Peter, and Niklas Rose. 2008. *Governing the Present: Administering Economic, Social and Political Life*. Malden: Polity Press.

Oliver, Denis. 1985. 'Reducing Suicide in Western Samoa', in F.X. Hezel, D.H. Rubinstein and G.M. White (eds), *Culture, Youth and Suicide in the Pacific: Papers from an East-West Center Conference*. Occasional Paper Series 25. Honolulu: Pacific Islands Studies Program, Center for Asian and Pacific Studies, University of Hawai'i at Mānoa, pp. 74–86.

Ragin, Charles C. 2014. *The Comparative Method: Moving beyond Qualitative and Quantitative Strategies*. Berkeley: University of California Press.

Redfield-Jamison, Kay. 1999. *Night Falls Fast: Understanding Suicide*. New York: Alfred A. Knopf.

Rubinstein, Donald H. 1983. 'Epidemic Suicide among Micronesian Adolescents', *Social Science and Medicine* 17(10): 657–65.

———. 1995. 'Love and Suffering: Adolescent Socialization and Suicide in Micronesia', *The Contemporary Pacific* 7(1): 21–53.

Schneidman, Edwin S. 1996. *The Suicidal Mind*. Oxford: Oxford University Press.

Schnegg, Michael. 2014. 'Anthropology and Comparison: Methodological Challenges and Tentative Solutions', *Zeitschrift für Ethnologie* 139(1): 55–72.

——— · 2019. 'The Life of Winds: Knowing the Namibian Weather from Someplace and from Noplace', *American Anthropologist* 121(4): 830–44.

Seeberg, Jens, and Lotte Meinert. 2015. 'Can Epidemics be Noncommunicable? Reflections on the Spread of "Noncommunicable" Diseases', *Medicine Anthropology Theory* 2(2): 54–71.

Staples, James, and Tom Widger. 2012. 'Situating Suicide as an Anthropological Problem: Ethnographic Approaches to Understanding Self-Harm and Self-Inflicted Death', *Culture, Medicine and Psychiatry* 36(4): 183–203.

Stevenson, Lisa. 2014. *Life beside Itself: Imagining Care in the Canadian Arctic*. Oakland: University of California Press.

Strathern, Marilyn. 1988. *The Gender of the Gift: Problems with Women and Problems with Society in Melanesia*. Berkeley: University of California Press.

Taylor, Charles. 1989. *The Sources of the Self: The Making of Modern Identity*. Cambridge, MA: Harvard University Press.

Va'a, Felise. 1982. 'Samoa's Youth Suicide Wave', *Pacific Islands Monthly* 53(7): 28–29. Retrieved 9 April 2015 from Google database.

Ward, Martha. 2004. *Nest in the Wind: Adventures in Anthropology on a Tropical Island*, 2nd edn. Long Grove, IL: Waveland Press.

Weisner, Thomas S., and Edward D. Lowe. 2004. 'Globalization, Childhood, and Psychological Anthropology', in C. Casey and R.B. Edgerton (eds), *A Companion to Psychological Anthropology: Modernity and Psychocultural Change*. Malden, MA: Blackwell Publishing, pp. 315–36.

Widger, Tom. 2015. *Suicide in Sri Lanka: The Anthropology of an Epidemic*, Kindle edn. London: Routledge.

Wilson, Catherine. 2014. 'Youth Suicides Sound Alarm across the Pacific'. Inter Press Service News Agency, 12 August. Retrieved 6 July 2016 from Google database.

Zigon, Jarrett. 2007. 'Moral Breakdown and the Ethical Demand: A Theoretical Framework for an Anthropology of Moralities', *Anthropological Theory* 7(2): 131–50.

Chapter 3
Haunted by the Future
Autism and the Spectre of Prison – Configuring Race and Disability in the African American Community

Cheryl Mattingly and Stephanie Keeney Parks

Introduction

This book asks: 'How do epidemics spread?' The pithy answer is 'through contagion'. This sounds merely tautological until you shift your gaze and attend not to diseases spread through infection but to social or 'noncommunicable' ones. As the editors point out, 'not all epidemics can be attributed to infection. A large part of the global burden of disease is due to so-called noncommunicable diseases'. Syndemics play a crucial role. 'Syndemics', following Singer et al. (2017), 'challenge[s] conventional historical understandings of diseases as distinct entities in nature, separate from other diseases and independent of social contexts'. The notion of syndemics allows us to take social contexts into consideration. It also highlights the pernicious results that can arise when multiple epidemics play out together, an especially prevalent phenomenon for populations living in impoverished conditions. Scholars emphasizing the role of political economy have led the way in examining how life conditions and health disparities influence contagions of both infectious and noncommunicable diseases (Farmer 2009;

Farmer et al. 2004; Nguyen and Peschard 2003; Seeberg and Meinert 2015).

In this chapter, we engage with epidemics and syndemics by considering the configuration of two such noncommunicable 'diseases'. More specifically, we investigate autism and the mass incarceration of the Black populations in the United States. The former is a category of intellectual difference and the latter is a rapidly increasing social epidemic afflicting minorities, especially Black communities, within the US. We consider autism – a mental health classification that has taken on epidemic proportions in recent decades within the US and even globally – as it intersects with the epidemic of mass imprisonment within the African American community. We identify how African Americans employ 'local epistemologies' to conceptualize the interconnection between the two. But we are most concerned with how African American parents of children (especially boys) at risk of diagnosis with autism spectrum disorder (ASD) *respond* to the threat of this syndemic. We explore the inoculating strategies they employ as they try to protect the *future* of their children from the life-threatening spectre of an adulthood characterized by chronic unemployment and potential incarceration.

Eluding the School-to-Prison Pipeline

Drawing on our individual fieldwork, we offer two case studies of boys who are considered to have ASD and their mothers' experiences with this diagnosis.[1] We should also mention that Stephanie is herself not only a PhD student in linguistic and medical anthropology but also an African American mother who has a young son with autism. While we do not include any autobiographical moments from her own experience, her richly informed lived knowledge helps to inform the analysis we offer. We attend, in particular, to two mothers' sustained efforts to prevent their children from being given an autistic label. In one case, Malcolm has been diagnosed with ASD by clinical and education specialists, but his mother (Autumn) rejects this diagnosis and moves him to school districts where she can avoid the categorization. In the second case, the child has eluded an ASD diagnosis only through the concerted efforts of his mother ('Dr Mom'), a trained psychologist who has developed elaborate strategies to prevent this, although she is convinced that he is, in fact, autistic. These two mothers are concerned not only to provide the best environment and educational support for their children's needs, but also to protect their children, as far as possible, from the pernicious stigma and impoverished life possibilities that so frequently accompany this diagnostic category for a child of colour. The figure of the incarcerated Black man looms as one such spectre.

But a puzzle emerges when we consider the response of these two mothers. As elaborated below, a wealth of data shows that African Americans have been systematically *underdiagnosed* with ASD. If health disparities for African Americans are visible as an underdiagnosis when it comes to autism, why are these two mothers so keen to avoid this classification? And why is it worth so much effort? What is so dangerous about it that they devote enormous energy to dodging it? The answer to these questions becomes apparent only when we treat an autism diagnosis in the Black community syndemically, that is, as one element in a configuration in which the epidemic of incarceration plays a pivotal role.

As we shall see, the evasive tactics of the two women are costly at a personal level. Both women labour diligently in forms of what might be called 'home-schooling', though home education looks quite different in the two cases. Their efforts speak to a common practice within the African American community in which the 'homeplace' is a crucial site of fugitive domestic efforts to defy (however quietly) an external world characterized by racialized power structures and stigmatizing forces (hooks 1990). The two mothers in our cases may struggle to create homeplaces that will protect their children, but there are very real limits and high personal tolls exacted by their strategic efforts.

The Contagion of Autism

Autism is a prime example of a non-contagious 'disease' whose rapid spread, both in the United States and globally, invites exploration of the social construction of biology. It has been marked as a diagnostic epidemic rather than a biological one. That is, there is no evidence that the *rise* in prevalence is related to any biological factors. There are no biological markers or environmental factors known to trigger symptoms and confirm a diagnosis (King and Bearman 2011). Even those who do not question that ASD has some kind of biological underpinnings attribute its rapid rise to recent shifts in categorization and the reorganizing of diagnostic criteria. Thus, Richard Grinker calls it an 'epidemic of discovery' (2007).

Autism has served as a notable exemplar of how new types of biosociality are developed. Powerful disability activist groups have arisen around it, influencing the direction of scientific research for treatment and cure as well as promoting the expansion of rights and services. Hacking (1999) has described it as a syndrome that is created through a 'looping effect' process in which expert decisions and the populations they designate and define work together to produce new identities (Rapp 2011; Silverman 2008). It is also a disorder that reveals the role of race and class in the production of a psychological category. Autism has been racially marked since its earliest presentation in 1943 (Grinker 2007; Grinker, Yeargin-Allsopp and Boyle 2011). It was famously blamed upon bad parenting, specifically the 'refrigerator mother', a term referring to educated, white, professional mothers (Bettelheim 1972; Kanner 1949; Liu, King and Bearman 2010). In the United States, autism is still far more frequently diagnosed in Euro-American and wealthier communities (Grinker 2007; King and Bearman 2011).

If autism is an epidemic, it is an uneven one. In the US, especially for African Americans, autism reveals the subtleties and local inflections of very dramatic health disparities along race and class lines in terms of delayed or non-diagnosis and lack of services. The comparatively lower rates of autism among African Americans, especially those living in poor areas, suggests a health disparity that shows up as *diminished prevalence* (Kogan et al. 2009; Merikangas et al. 2010; Silverman 2012). Children from an ethnic or racial minority group are more likely to experience delayed diagnosis (Mandell et al. 2002; Overton, Fielding and de Alba 2007). This does not mean that these children are 'escaping' a mental health diagnosis. Rather, they are being diagnosed *differently*. African American children are 2.6 times *less* likely than Anglo-American children to receive an autism diagnosis on their first clinical visit and three times *more* likely to be given conduct or adjustment disorder diagnoses which are more stigmatizing and have fewer services attached (Mandell et al. 2007, 2009).

How might we think about this as a contagion? The dramatic health disparities surrounding it also suggest the importance of investigating how life conditions (for example, one's social, racial and economic status) influence its spread – that is, when and under what circumstances a cluster of symptoms and behaviours warrants an ASD diagnosis. What becomes clear is that the relatively slower spread of the diagnosis among African Americans is linked not to better life situations (as with so many diagnoses) but to worse ones. If this is the case – to return to the central puzzle of this chapter – why are the two mothers not advocating for their children to get the (expensive) educational and clinical services that law mandates children with this diagnosis should receive? This is not a simple case of poverty. It is precisely *because* they are both middle class and their children live in relatively well-funded public schools that an ASD diagnosis and special education services have been proffered. If they lived in more impoverished school districts, this option would not even be available.

It is only by thinking configurationally, and syndemically, that these puzzles can be unravelled.

The Contagion of Prison

Within the United States, the epidemic of mass incarceration for Black people starts as early as a child's entrance into the school system, especially for those placed into special education. In one study completed by the Pew Research Center and the National Association for the Advancement of Colored People (NAACP), the impact of mass incarceration has created an increase from five hundred thousand prisoners to over two million since the 1980s. The significant rise in incarceration coincides with the racist policies of Ronald Reagan's 'war on drugs' that began in that decade, followed by the impact of the Clinton administration and their characterization of Black males as 'super predators'. Black adults are incarcerated at five times the rate of white adults, making up 34 per cent of the prison population, although they constitute only 13 per cent of the total US population (NAACP n.d.a; Pew Research Center 2013).

A common statistic cited by Black Americans is that one in three Black boys will be incarcerated in their lifetimes, a number that is also supported by the NAACP (n.d.a). Education scholars have noted that special education for Black children in the United States serves as a 'pipeline' to future incarceration. Rather than special education functioning as a haven of protection and support for students with disabilities, it acts as a 'playground' for the school-to-prison pipeline (Powell and Keeney Parks forthcoming; Wald and Losen 2003). The threat of future imprisonment is particularly ominous for Black children because of their overidentification and placement in special education as they acquire a diffuse range of cognitive and behavioural disability and deficit labels. Statistically speaking, this widespread school segregation practice results in lifetime negative outcomes for Black students, including significantly higher numbers of incarcerations when compared to white peers.

Black parents, as illustrated by Autumn and Dr Mom, are attuned to the future possibilities that their children face. They are also aware that processes leading to incarceration begin early in their children's lives and that school plays a decisive role. Racism displayed by educators in the US public school system is well documented in the disproportionate adverse disciplinary actions such as school suspension of Black students, especially those in special education. In fact, Black students in special education constitute the largest portion of students suspended annually. During the school years 2014–16, Black students with disabilities were suspended at a rate so high that on average they lost upwards of seventy [additional] days of school instruction when compared to their white disabled peers (Erevelles 2014; Losen 2018; Noguera 2003). Black males experience the highest rates of school suspension with a rate of 17.6 per cent compared to white males at a rate of 3.4 per cent (National Center of Education Statistics, February 2019).[2] Youth of colour are also disproportionately placed in juvenile detention facilities, a particularly direct route into the adult prison system as children age out of juvenile institutions. The American Civil Liberties Union (ACLU) found that this contributed to 'a disturbing national trend wherein children are funneled out of public schools and into carceral systems' (ACLU 2014).

Haunted by the Future

Thus far, we have offered an array of statistics to depict these epidemics. Statistics lead to puzzles – why do these mothers resist a diagnosis that African Americans have been comparatively deprived of?

And they suggest provisional answers. School in general, and special education in particular, turns out to hold special threats for a high percentage of Black children, especially those with disabilities. When we turn to our two ethnographic cases, these statistics do not simply come to life as they are concretely lived, in the manner of putting flesh on abstract figures and generalizations. The cases offer a nuance that has conceptual implications, suggesting other directions for thought and analysis. Taken together, they provide a kind of narrative anthropological extension of the syndemics theory originally developed by Singer and colleagues. They ask us to think in terms of metaphors and narratives of disease and pathology at the level of cultural imagination rather than merely epidemiologically. The cases also consider how a syndemic is lived and experienced. A syndemic – as experienced – is not only about suffering (though it is that). It is also about response, about action. The two mothers and their children who serve as the key protagonists of this chapter are more than recipients of structural violence. The mothers undertake strenuous projects of care to ameliorate its effects, including tangible effects that have already occurred and future effects they can foresee and attempt to ward off.

Although we do not elaborate a phenomenological approach in this chapter, we attend to experience on multiple fronts. We adopt a first-person approach that is a hallmark of phenomenological investigation. This does not mean, as is sometimes supposed, that we are focused on the single experiencing individual. Rather, we assume that the most direct route to investigating the world (in this case, a syndemic) is through an inquiry into how it is experienced, perceived, responded to. As feminist phenomenologist Salamon nicely puts it, the 'first-person experience is the zero point of phenomenology ... Despite its first-person vantage point ... phenomenology is advocating neither subjectivism nor solipsism. There is no perception without a subject but there is no subject without a world' (2018: 16). The large structural forces that impinge upon entire populations, the world at an aggregate level, emerge with stark clarity as lived by particular bodies in particular situations. This is what our chapter seeks to expose.

The title of our chapter also suggests another generative direction for investigating this syndemic: the concept of hauntology. Hauntology was coined by Derrida (1994), developed sociologically by Avery Gordon (2008), and in anthropology by Byron Good (2012, 2019), Maria Louw (2018) and others. Hauntology directs us to think not just historically, but in terms of the return of apparitional forms from buried pasts. Toni Morrison's brilliant novel *Beloved* (1987) was a key inspiration for Gordon, as it has been for a host of Black studies scholars. Situated historically at the end of the period of slavery in the United States, one of *Beloved*'s key protagonists is, in fact, a child who returns to haunt her family. The ghost forces an agonizing family process of 'rememory' (in Morrison's famous term) of violence born from slavery. Black studies scholars have often called upon Morrison's *Beloved*, thinking with ghosts as they develop rich analytics for imagining how to live 'in the wake of slavery, in slavery's afterlives', as Sharpe puts it (2016: 18; see also Hartman 1997; Spillers 2003).

It is beyond the scope of this chapter to dig more deeply into this provocative line of thought, but a spectral vocabulary reminds us to consider the long histories that create syndemics such as the one we explore. Hauntological investigations reveal how histories of trauma are lived, how traumas may be hidden or passed over, only to make their restless appearance as so many unhappy ghosts. Ghosts may be real, of course (Hollan 2019). But might we even think of diagnostic categories in ghostly terms?

There is a history to the syndemic we explore but it is not the mere accidental history of one unfortunate moment in time or state of affairs. Rather, this syndemic merely refigures antiblack racial trauma in yet another guise. Autism, in other words, is not so much the *cause* of a new kind of danger or threat, but another vehicle which, when affixed to Black children (especially boys), generates danger. The ghost that truly haunts is not the disability category itself but the carceral space it beckons. And beyond that, the ghost of racial trauma, still very much alive, originating some five hundred years ago with the founding of the 'New World' as a colonial project. To live historically, if one belongs to a community in danger, as African Americans do, is to live with trauma as it is passed down, relived, and recast in new forms over generations. To be haunted is not only to be plagued by the restless activity of unhappy ghosts, by a past that is not dead, but to be confronted with a future menaced by a trauma not yet lived, and which one neglects at one's peril (Derrida 1994; Good 2019; Gordon 2008; Lincoln and Lincoln 2015).

Malcolm: A Category and a Mother in Dialogue

Cheryl first met Autumn and her son Malcolm early in 2002. They joined a research study of African American families raising children with chronic illnesses and severe disabilities in the Los Angeles area. The longitudinal ethnographic study, which is described in more detail elsewhere (see especially Mattingly 2010) began in 1997 and ended (officially) in 2011. It involved a large research team who followed a total of fifty families to clinical encounters, observing and videotaping many of those encounters, and following children to home, school and community events. Families directed us to accompany them to those social events and spaces they deemed significant for their children.

At the time Autumn and Malcolm entered the study, Malcolm was five years old. He had been diagnosed with a range of neurological, sensory and behavioural disorders, including, at times, autism spectrum disorder. He was, as one neurologist told Autumn, 'on the spectrum'. She finds this diagnosis particularly contagious and pernicious, unlike some of the other diagnoses offered by clinicians over the years. At two-and-a-half, Malcolm was diagnosed with a delay in speech attributed to complete blockage in one ear and hearing loss. This hearing loss was corrected surgically but the clinicians who tested him for hearing also began to notice other problems – increased activity, decreased attention span – and thus began an array of disability labels, including autism. Autumn did not discard all disability labels, but this was one she adamantly refused. It was not a category she would allow her son to catch. She describes an early conversation with a neurologist and school specialists whom she confronted: 'Because I said, *look* at him. He is not autistic'. The clinicians were puzzled by what they saw as her obstinacy. 'I guess she's in denial', one therapist remarked. 'I don't know why she's being so rigid about this.'

Her rejection of autism involves a long and tortuous process of moving Malcolm from school to school and community to community in an effort to evade its grasp. As noted earlier, from a structural vantage point, the autism diagnosis is not contagious *enough* for African American children; they are systematically underdiagnosed and underserved. But Autumn responds to the diagnosis as though it were a pernicious infection from which she must flee to protect her son. How might we explain this? In one of the early interviews with her, she gives a sense of why she felt compelled to run from it. She depicts the kind of conversation she anticipates if she tells people that her son has autism. 'Ohhh', her imagined interlocutor responds, in a disinterested voice, followed by silence, an evident end to the conversation. She concludes: 'You know, where as most people don't understand autism but they think they do'. Because it has become familiar in popular imagination, people think they know about it. Instead of being curious to get to know her son, people will misunderstand and dismiss him. They presume his slow speech and halting words reflect a slow mind. But this, she firmly insists, is not her son.

A phenomenological perspective alerts us that what Autumn is describing is a *form of experience* that endangers her son. It is an inter-relational space characterized by lack of curiosity and dismissal, one where her son has no visibility or, more precisely, is visible only as a member of a stigmatized category – a child with mental handicaps. The experience of dismissal she describes is very dangerous; it has the potential to 'infect' her son by placing him in situations in which he actively learns to – in her words – 'become nothing'. Cheryl first heard her speak of this kind of becoming when he was only six years old, giving a complex temporality to her words: 'I did not raise him to become nothing'. She speaks as though he is already grown, and she is looking backward into the past. She is 'always already' living a future within that present moment. Autism is no longer a DSM category into which her son is placed by psychology and neurology experts. Rather it is merely one expression, one name, for a possible future – a becoming that she must guard against. It is also shapeshifting; it can take many social forms, including, she discovers, the life of street 'gangstas'.

Autumn's words offer a phenomenological resonance, a meditation on lived time, and also a cultural resonance. Her reference to this spectre of 'nothing' carries particular weight culturally and linguistically within the African American speech community. More specifically, she signifies. Signifying is a common feature of African American discourse (Abrahams 1963; Kochman 1969; Mitchell-Kernan 1971, 1972; Smitherman 1973, 1977) and is 'a means to encode messages or meaning in natural conversations, usually involving an element of indirection' (Alim 2005: 183). When Autumn uses the phrase 'becoming nothing', she offers a culturally salient linguistic 'short hand' that identifies the complicated and problematic position of a Black disabled male in American society. Autumn's phrasing also employs code switching as she describes her son's situation to white researchers. Code switching, another common feature of African American conversational style, is a form of 'verbal dexterity' (Alim, Smitherman and Dyson 2012; Baugh 2003; Bucholtz 2012; Harness-Goodwin and Alim 2010; Morgan 1994; Smitherman 1977, 1999, 2000). In Autumn's words, the signifier 'becoming nothing' is a code-switched version of the more typical 'that n— ain't nothin'.

In what follows, Autumn offers two stories that indicate how 'becoming nothing' emerges as a contaminating experience of misrecognition in which race, disability and gender are dangerously intertwined. 'Becoming nothing' could be understood as a 'local epistemology' or even an 'emic phenomenology', a common phrase in the African American community. In Autumn's case, it also names a temporally complex form of intersubjective experience that manifests differently in different situations and bears upon Malcolm's future self. When Malcolm's autism diagnosis threatens to plunge him into a life of 'becoming nothing' because he is a 'boy of colour', as his mother says, his plight reveals intersectionality as a lived danger of potentiality. We see the configuration of race, gender and disability poised to shape a future of being 'nothing'.

Autism thus poses both a present danger and a future threat. There is no question in her mind that race factors in the apparent inability of clinical and educational experts to recognize her son's cognitive complexity, his intellectual talents, the sheer mystery of his mental life. In the following exchange, in a family group meeting that was part of the research project, Autumn talks with Tanya (an African American mother who has a child with cerebral palsy) about the problem of Malcolm getting negative labels attached to him. Being African American, Autumn believes, makes disability labels more lethal.

> Autumn: Part of the problem is also that I think that they look at children of colour when they have disabilities, that its more, 'oh, no, you know, they can't be helped' kind of thing.
> Tanya: [nodding her head in agreement] Yeah.

Autumn: And I ran into that this summer, and I was just like, sort of blind-sided with it. Ran into that this summer with summer school.

Autumn then offers a detailed account of how she was 'blind-sided' by the teacher in her child's summer school programme. This was a programme that combined children from regular education with those in special education and the summer school teacher who was not familiar with Malcolm. Autumn is stunned by the way he becomes a problem for the teacher through what she believes to be the teacher's own incompetence. She faults the teacher not only for actually creating a situation in which her son comes to be seen as the problem, but the fact that the school did not inform her that this problem was occurring so that she could intervene. Autumn said that her child's 'one on one' (an assistant whose job is to work with an individual child within the classroom) was sending notes home with Malcolm each day with 'happy faces' (meaning that he is doing well) 'because he *responds* to happy faces, okay? So we're getting this every day'. This leads Autumn to assume that Malcolm is doing fine in school until one day she gets a note from the teacher to call – always an ominous sign.

Autumn: Well I get a note on that sheet, 'Please call the teacher'. Okay, so I called, left a message. She didn't call me back. So the next week I went to the school, [the teacher tells her] 'Oh, I'm glad you came. And I'm really concerned'.

Autumn recounts her internal response to this ('And I'm like, first of all you didn't call me back, so how concerned could you be?') as well as the exchange she and the teacher had. 'And, so then she's sitting there and she's talking. "I'm really concerned about your child. He's belligerent. He has to sit at a table all by himself. He has to do this". I'm saying, "Wait, wait, you talking about my son?" And I'm saying, "Wait, wait, wait. My son you're talking about? Malcolm?"'

Autumn sets up another meeting when Malcolm's assistant can also attend so they can talk this through. The assistant confirms, in milder language, what the teacher has reported. Autumn recounts the assistant's words: '"He's physical and he's big. He doesn't realize how strong he is ... I'm scared for the other children". And on and on'. Tanya interrupts. 'Oh, brother.' Autumn continues her story, conveying her shocked reaction as she wonders, 'What is going on here?' She gets an answer sometime later. She finds evidence of how

Malcolm is being handled by the teacher and assistant such that this 'belligerence' is created through their problematic interaction.

> Autumn: And, so then, I saw it when I was talking to her [the teacher] individually, and Malcolm was off playing. And he would do something [that he should not be doing]. And I would say [*she makes her voice soft*] 'Okay, you need to clean that up'. And right behind me, she's [*Autumn shifts her tone, becoming annoyed and urgent*] 'Okay *you* need to get that cleaned up!'

Autumn brought this up at a subsequent meeting with the teacher: 'And so then, I told her at the other meeting when the assistant was there, I said, "You know what? I see him responding to your frustration, Okay?" "Oh, I'm not, I don't show him that." I said, "You're showing it in front of me. I know he feels it, and he's pushing that button because he feels it". You know, and I told her at that meeting, I said, "You know, people do mistake children with disabilities for – that they also have mental deficiencies, okay?" I said, "My son is very bright. He just doesn't sit still long, okay?"'

> Tanya: [*adds*] They automatically attach a label to the child.
> Autumn: [*nods her head*] Right.
> Tanya: Or they say, okay – well I've gotten this too – 'Well, what did you, did you take drugs when you were...'
> Group: [*responds to this*] Oooh! Oh, goodness.
> Autumn: It's like, don't take me there. [*laughter*]
> Tanya: Already a negative, negative.
> Autumn: [*overlaps*] And then they label. Like I said, they label your child. And they're very quick to say, 'First of all, he's an African American child. So therefore, they're more aggressive anyhow'. [*Tanya nods in agreement*] You know, and along those lines.

In her coda to the summer school story, Autumn emphasizes the role of race in aiding this 'quickness' with labels and the logic of these professional experts. Being African American is not just part of the figure – it is 'first of all'. Her child is submerged into a third person, African American 'they' who are 'more aggressive'. In this exchange the two mothers object that when disability labels intersect with a race category like African American, children are known before they have a chance to reveal themselves. The image of the difficult, potentially violent Black male thoroughly configures Malcolm's encounters at school. Teachers 'pre-understand'

Malcolm, to put it in hermeneutic terms, in ways that blind them to how their own behaviours and expectations help create the very child they label in this damaging way. In this situation, 'becoming nothing' manifests itself in the hazardous form: 'problem student'. As a form of experience, it speaks to more than mere mislabelling, for it creates the very reality that it names. Malcolm responds to the teacher by becoming, in fact, difficult, consciously 'pushing her buttons'. He *becomes* a problem student.

The Contagion of a Syndemic: Touched by 'Gangsta' Life

Meinert and Seeberg (this volume) note that when it comes to non-communicable diseases, 'contagion' is often used metaphorically. But they are after something else, how even such noncommunicable conditions can be, quite literally, contagious. Autumn offers an especially compelling account of how her son began to catch the 'disease' of nothingness. When Malcolm turned seven, she relocated so that she could enrol him in a new school district where they have small classrooms for children with behavioural problems. But to her horror, her son 'started picking up *very bad* habits. That's when he started learning how to cuss. You know? Started saying "Wanna be a gangsta, wanna live on the street". And I'm like, "You're only seven years old! *Seven!*"' She found out that the classroom consisted of boys 'that were being *kicked* out of their schools. Like incorrigibles, you know? This was the kind of school that they were gonna stay in. Rather than, it being a helping point in moving on'.

Malcolm begins to imitate the boys whose lives he admires. 'And there he perfected his cussing', she said. 'He went from, you know, very interested in dinosaurs and everything – wanting to be a palaeontologist – to wanting to be a gangsta.' She shakes her head in sorrow. 'His aspirations sunk low.' Her words might be heard as a condemnation of the 'incorrigible' children Malcolm meets at school and their 'gangsta life'. Certainly, she is not celebrating the richness of gang culture or recognizing its possibilities for becoming; joining a gang is assuredly not the future she wants for her son. However, her words suggest a more subtle condemnation directed not at the children but at a school which, rather than being a 'helping point' for children 'in moving on' is a dead end, the kind of school that children will 'stay in'. As a form of experience, 'becoming nothing' now manifests itself as a trap that erases the possibility for movement at all. Or, put differently, it is a form of life in which, Autumn's story suggests, becoming is no longer possible.

Thinking with the language of the 'syndemic', we can see how autism emerges as a presence that keeps mutating as a child comes into contact with a school situation in which his fellow classmates are being funnelled into lives that will almost surely lead them into prison. In order to avoid this contagious school situation, Autumn flees yet again. Although Autumn has followed the advice of a Special Education Director whom she trusted and who persuaded her that this programme would be a better fit for her son, she holds herself accountable for this error in judgement – for her own blindness. Shaken, she pulls Malcolm out and enrols him in a private, religious school that has no special education services, an inadequate 'best good' where he will no longer be eligible for the speech therapy that she knows he needs.

'Dr Mom': Confronting the Danger of an Autism Diagnosis

Our second case centres around Dr Rosa Smith and her son Isaac. It comes from research undertaken by Stephanie as part of her master's thesis during the year 2016–17. Dr Smith was initially not a participant in Stephanie's research project, but rather a clinical expert and cultural insider as a Black woman who is also a behavioural psychologist specializing in autism. She is both clinician and faculty member at a prominent university. During one of many conversations, Dr Smith told Stephanie about her son and her own personal experience parenting a special needs child. Stephanie had not previously been aware of her son's diagnosis. While Dr Smith disclosed her own assessment of her child Isaac to Stephanie, she had publicly refused to have her child receive this diagnosis.[3]

How does Dr Smith elude the category of ASD? She draws on her own expertise in her interactions with school and clinical professionals to present her child as having disabilities more fitting for a diagnosis she deems less threatening – namely attention deficit hyperactivity disorder (ADHD). 'I know what to say.' That is how Dr Smith explained how she was able to access a diagnosis of ADHD for her child. When Stephanie asked why she opted for an ADHD classification, she replied: 'What is a diagnosis that we can live with, that is a very normal one to have? Let's go with that one'.

Dr Smith is acutely aware that she is misguiding her child's paediatricians and teachers, saying:

> When it comes to our son, we know he is different and that there is clearly something delayed, but we [Dr Smith and her spouse], well we just said 'we'll just handle things as they come to us'. And you know, the school, well the school sees him as a kid that can't or won't focus. I don't really know how intentional all of our responses really were, but we did intentionally get him diagnosed with ADHD, first with the school – we needed it for state testing – and then I went to the paediatrician. You know, I know how it all works, I know what to say.

At the time of Stephanie's initial encounters with Dr Smith, Isaac was in elementary school, and he was struggling. His grades were low, and his sensory processing was making everyday tasks like eating and hair brushing at best a fight and at worst nearly impossible. He was having a hard time connecting to his classmates and often did not feel like he 'fit in' or had friends. Isaac also showed signs of difficulty in his executive planning, making learning and processing information difficult. These difficulties were not new, but rather had been a lifelong struggle for Isaac, leading Rosa to believe that her son did indeed have autism.

Rosa expresses her ideals of a good life for her child in the language of normalcy. She strives for a 'more normal', as she puts it. She rejects an ASD label because she is convinced it will constrict her child's future possibilities in ways she will not accept. She fears it will preclude him from engaging in a socially significant or 'more normal' life experience such as college. But why, specifically, is an ASD label so pernicious, from her perspective, in a way that ADHD is not? For her, the answer lies in an institutional configuration within the US school system. For Dr Smith and her husband, an 'accurate' diagnosis is not tied to what is clinically accurate as, for example, defined by the Diagnostic and Statistical Manual of Mental Disorders, 5th Edition (DSM5) (the official diagnostic manual for mental health disorders produced by the American Medical Association). Rather, an accurate diagnosis is tied to keeping their child safe when he is in environments outside his home, most notably the education system. But how does shaping the language of her son's diagnosis to reflect ADHD versus autism keep her son safe?

This is not immediately obvious. Her efforts to help her son acquire an ADHD diagnosis also endanger him because the relative mildness of this category encourages teachers to construe some of Isaac's more severe challenges not as disability related but as behavioural problems that he could control better. As Dr Smith states, the school sees her child as a kid who 'can't or won't focus'. These are words that index ideas about Black boys in a very particular way, suggesting that children so designated may be wilfully not participating in school. While this is the very kind of characterization that has so often led to Black children being underdiagnosed for autism, it is a mischaracterization Dr Smith uses to her advantage. The teachers' readiness to see her son as someone who 'can't or won't focus' (the 'won't' blurring the 'can't') provides necessary protection within the school system. Dr Smith believes she is able to persuade them of the (clinically inaccurate) ADHD diagnosis by 'knowing what to say' because she can obliquely refer to commonly held racialized ideologies of 'can't or won't' that surround Black males in white public spaces. In other words, Dr Smith uses to advantage the racial figure of the belligerent Black boy that helps to produce systemic underdiagnosis of autism in children of colour. Dr Smith's strategic appropriation of a misdiagnosis to protect her child reveals the nuanced ways in which families are trying to navigate configuring forces that lead to unwanted outcomes for their children. But what, specifically, makes autism so dangerous as a diagnostic category that she is willing to risk her son's stigmatization as a disruptive, unruly Black child? In short: the special education classroom.

In Dr Smith's home state, a diagnosis of ADHD allows a child to gain access to resources such as alternative testing, private testing rooms (where a child can focus without the distraction of a regular classroom), and extra time to complete the test. Services may also include one-on-one teaching aide supports. These are all imperative supports for a child like Isaac, especially when he must undergo state mandated testing. State tests are used to place children into specific types of classrooms, most notably special education versus general education classrooms, and to help identify which children get access to higher-quality education such as advanced science, math, and reading classes. When Stephanie asked Dr Smith about her child having special education supports, she said, 'If I thought special education would serve him, then I would say "yes, give him that autism diagnosis", but I promise you, I will homeschool him. The data on special education is so bad'.

Federal documents such as the 504 and IEP (Individual Education Plan) are documents mandated by the Individuals with Disabilities Education Act (IDEA) as a means of outlining what types of supports a school will provide for a child who has been identified by the education system as having a disability. Dr Smith has managed to ensure that her son has a '504' and not an 'IEP' evaluation.

> Oh, he has a 504 and we are giving them hella trouble now. We are in a school that is 98 per cent white, that's why we are trying to keep these teachers in check. [She shakes her head in a mixture of annoyance and disgust.] These people call me by my first name, I am always respectful of them, calling his teacher Mrs Song, by her title. I mean we are not friends, why can't she call me 'Mrs'? Why do I have to respect her, and she doesn't recognize me? I am a behavioural psychologist; my title is Dr.

In Dr Smith's state, the 504 is used with 'less severe' children, such as those with ADHD. The 504 is often used to protect placement in general education classrooms and provide supports such as those described earlier. If Isaac were viewed by the state as more profoundly affected by his disability, he would be unable to 'fly under the radar'. If Isaac were subjected to an IEP, an Individual Education Plan, this would involve consultation with educators, school psychologists and possibly therapists and it would very likely dictate that he would be segregated out into a self-contained special education classroom. With an ADHD diagnosis, he will continue to be 'mainstreamed' into regular education classes. So long as Dr Smith can 'say the right thing', she can protect him from the level of stigma and the systemic problems that an autism diagnosis would create. She declares emphatically: 'I can't go the special ed route, not until I have to, and I still don't have to'.

Dr Smith leverages her knowledge about autism, racialized stereotypes, and data concerning abysmal outcomes for Black males in special education to gain access to a 'diagnosis that we can live with and looks more normal'. Her efforts reveal how the social contagion of autism has a much bigger impact than just the labelling of her son. Autism is also contagious to those around him because it will so profoundly change the expectation of his teachers. Their downgraded expectations of his abilities will, in turn, influence how he is able to engage in the educational environment. Autumn's story of Malcolm's teacher offers a potent example of the powerful effect of expectations in producing what they anticipate. Several decades ago, McDermott's wonderful essay 'The Acquisition of a Child by a Learning Disability' offered a seminal ethnographic depiction of this phenomenon in the world of American special education.

As Dr Smith puts it, when teachers engage with children who have been labelled with disabilities such as autism, they 'lower the bar'. 'Lowering the bar' means that her child would not be held to the same standards as his typically developing peers. She said, 'I know how people behave and how they reinforce behaviours … this is part of the problem with labels, the bar drops. They would lower their expectations of my child; I have seen studies that show how detrimental that can be for students when they have teachers that see them [the students] as less intelligent'. To combat this, Dr Smith finds ways to 'lie' or 'game the system'. She even once told her son's teacher that he had tested as 'gifted', she admits laughingly, with some embarrassment. 'I even once lied to a teacher telling them that my son had tested as gifted.' She explains: 'I have to game the system. I *have* to game the system. I don't know how long this will last, how long he will fly under the radar. But for now, it's working'.

Inoculating Responses: Homeplace

The Black feminist bell hooks (1990) describes 'homeplace' as a safe space where Black families can escape from the world. She also identifies 'homeplace' as a site of resistance where female parental figures do the work of teaching the next generation how to become Black people and how to stay safe in the outside white world. 'In our young minds houses belonged to women, were their special domain, not as property, but as places where all that truly mattered in life took place – the warmth and comfort of shelter, the feeding of our bodies, the nursing of our souls. There we learned dignity, integrity of being; there we learned to have faith. The folks who made this life possible, who were our primary guides and teachers, were black women' (hooks 1990: 41–42). For Autumn and Dr Smith, home provides the only truly safe haven while school, even if necessary and in some ways beneficial, is a continual threat, including their sons' exposure to racist labels and dismissals. They each cultivate homeplaces that can offer their sons inoculation against the dangerous threats of stigma, dismissal, exposure to low educational expectations or even a kind of waiting room for a future life in prison. Each of them recognizes that school itself – including 'regular ed' – does not work for their children; it does not provide a learning environment in which their children can actually learn. Thus, both are concerned to provide homes that offer learning environments. But they cultivate very different kinds of home experiences for their children. These differences are at least partly attributable to the personal and cultural resources they can bring to bear in providing care.

Unlike Autumn, Dr Smith is capable of providing the necessary and expensive therapy within her home. This eliminates the problem of finding a school, moving her family or navigating outside resources.

> Look, my take is this and this is just how I feel comfortable. School, school is a social institution. [She recounts imagined instructions to her son.] You go there and you socialize. And all of your school work – 'I will do this with you at home. I will tell you, I will teach what you need to know at home'. Because the school fuckin' can't. And yup, 'You just go to school and you have a good time. And you come home and work'.

According to Dr Smith, she has just 'flipped it', meaning that she has transposed the space, flipped the script. Instead of school being the place of learning, it has now become a social space. Instead of home being a space of play, the project of learning is now taking place within the home. This home project is extensive, even exhaustive, and she describes it in some detail:

> I am always trying to be mindful of my support of him [using Applied Behaviour Analysis], making sure it's not heavy handedness. It's all about teaching process, how do I focus on teaching him how to focus. I will stop [providing in home supports] when he doesn't respond to, when he becomes unresponsive to the support I provide, then I will stop. So I am doing this to have him keep pace [with his school age peers].

When thinking about her son and his needs, the homeplace is where she can teach him skills so that he can participate in the outside white world.

> Dr Smith: I know we are adequately servicing him at home, but I know that as he grows older and demands get greater ... Every morning I put the food in his mouth [alluding to a feeding disorder commonly associated with children that have autism].
> Stephanie: In your home you are doing everything, like in the clinic ABA, including feeding?
> Dr Smith: We're just doing everything. We were up until 10 last night doing homework, and it's not even like homework, it's that we also enrolled him in Kumon [outside tutoring company] which does reading and math, so um, we do that. Every night we do a reading packet, we do a math packet. He reads out loud to his dad for twenty minutes and um then we do whatever school work he has on top of that ... every single night.
> Stephanie: Is he academically close to his peers?
> Dr Smith: Yup and that is where we are working to keep him. That is exactly what we are trying to maintain. So all of his teachers are just convinced that he just has ADHD and that this is a focus or behaviour problem and that he is really smart and I am like 'ok, that sounds great'. So my husband asked me, 'what are you gonna do when he comes home with letter grades and he is a C student?' I said, 'Imma keep supporting him 'cause without that, he would be an F student, right?' I mean we are just scraping by and I am not going to lie to you, we are just trying to keep people's perceptions where I want them of him so they don't treat him differently and so that they can keep their expectations high so I can sneakily come behind him and give him supports to get there. That's all I am doing.

While Autumn does not have the professional skills or knowledge of the school system to accomplish what Dr Smith can do at home for her son, she brings other resources to bear. She sees Malcolm as a child rich in imagination and she exploits this capability at home, where she tries to surround him with the kinds of activities that call upon his curiosity. One simple example will suffice, a time during his earlier years (from six to about nine) when he was obsessed with dinosaurs. The extent to which Malcolm inhabited a prehistoric world became especially evident when you visited his bedroom, in which there were shelves and shelves of dinosaurs. Plastic ones, soft fabric ones that can be cuddled at night, dangerous ones showing their sharp teeth. This world materializes not only in Malcolm's room but in his treasured DVD collection, which includes three movies about dinosaurs that he watches again and again. On one visit by a member of the research team, Jeannie Gaines, he shows her one of his three favourite films, *Big Al*, and tries to entice her into a time, some 230 million years ago, when Big Al roamed the earth, a time currently inhabited by Malcolm.

We include a few minutes of this visit in Malcolm's room where Jeannie and Autumn are talking, as Jeannie tries to interview Autumn, but where Malcolm insistently intervenes, trying to draw Jeannie into the world where Big Al (and Malcolm) live. In this interlude, Jeannie is asking Autumn some questions about Malcolm's physical development ('Has he lost any teeth yet?'), while Malcolm jumps up and down on his bed. He has been showing Jeannie his treasure house of dinosaurs and he now wants to show her one of his favourite films. He introduces this possibility in the following way.

> Malcolm: [*jumping on his bed*] I'm a…
> JG: [*interrupts to ask Autumn*] No tooth fairy experiences or?
> Malcolm: …fossil.
> Autumn: [*replying to Jeannie*] No, not yet.
> Malcolm: [*Malcolm continues jumping on his bed*] I'm a fossil.
> Autumn: [*turning to Malcolm*] You're a fossil?
> Malcolm: I don't have these [mumbled] bones. Rawr. [*He stops jumping and points to his stomach*].
> Autumn: [*to Jeannie*] When he tells you, when he recites a story he does it so fast that if you don't know what he's talking about it's like what, what, what is he saying? But because I know most of them.

As Autumn and Jeannie continue talking, Malcolm gets off the bed, slithers to the ground in the manner of a large lizard and makes his way to Jeannie. He opens his mouth wide, growls, roars and pretends to bite her feet. 'Oh no!' she exclaims in mock fear. 'Ouchy, ouchy. My toe's hurting.' After a few minutes more, as Jeannie and August carry on their conversation, Malcolm has the idea of showing *Big Al*. Autumn obligingly puts it into the DVD player, and it begins to play. 'There', Malcolm says to Jeannie, pointing at the movie that has just come on. 'What is this we're gonna watch?' Jeannie asks. Malcolm mumbles, 'we'll watch that one'. Autumn, prompting him asks, 'What is it called?' Malcolm responds, 'It's called Big Al'. Autumn concurs, 'Big Al, yes'.

Jeannie begins another conversation with Autumn about when Malcolm was little. Autumn sometimes redirects the conversation back to the film and Malcolm also tries to direct attention back into the story, narrating parts he finds especially fascinating. He names different dinosaurs as they come into view, pointing to the screen to show Jeannie. 'The stegosaurus', he says. Autumn replies, 'Uh-oh. What is he– what is he doing?' in reference to the dinosaur he pointed out. Malcolm then tells them that he runs around. Malcolm illustrates the dinosaur's life, roaring. And he continues to point out the other dinosaurs that roam the screen, naming them effortlessly.

> Malcolm: The ploticus. [*he points*] The ploticus. Mommy, mommy, mommy. The ploticus.
> Autumn: The ploticus. Yes.
> Malcolm: Apatosaurus.
> Autumn: Apatosaurus, very good.

Malcolm watches, entranced, as the apatosaurus stomps across, stretching its long neck and shaking the ground beneath his feet. 'Whoa', Malcolm says, awed. Malcolm has learned how to play in these worlds. They have provided experiences for him in the strongest sense – places where 'something happens'. In them, he also becomes a something, a shark, a fossil. He tries to solicit others to join him there. He is most successful with his mother, who knows the same stories. Autumn finds herself 'following' Malcolm through his own journeys into these imaginative universes. She helps to facilitate his entry into these worlds through her efforts to find out what interests him. To understand her son, she must go through a kind of detour into the culturally crafted worlds where sharks, dinosaurs and other 'monsters' live. All those who want to understand Malcolm must also find their way into these worlds in order to find him.

The Cost of Inoculation and the Limits of the Homeplace

Although homeplaces like those that Dr Smith and Autumn create provide powerful sites of learning, connection and even resistance for African American children, the work of cultivating them demands a high price from the women who are largely or solely responsible. In the case of Autumn and Dr Smith, this is exacerbated by the fact that both have full-time positions outside the home, which means that they must, in effect, carry out two full-time jobs.

> Dr Smith: It's hard, this is all on me, that's the hardest part. So like if things don't go well then it happened because, well whatever, it's on me. Like I am never doing enough, like I shouldn't be working, shouldn't be doing this or that or having this conversation, I should be doing his stuff right now. So...

Both mothers find that there is a guilt associated with creating a lifeworld where their children can thrive and become more than 'nothing'. Black feminists have given critical attention to costs associated with this task of creating homeplaces. It may be possible and indeed necessary to provide this kind of home care in order to protect Black children (with or without disabilities), but it comes with a cost. Historically, there have been high expectations within the African American community that women cultivate nurturing and protective homes even as they also hold down full-time jobs. The culturally iconic ideal of being a 'superstrong black woman' carries a price of never being good enough. Dr Mom and Autumn exemplify this in several ways, even though Dr Mom (unlike Autumn) is married. Both are full-time professionals whose work creates an uneasy relationship between being a 'good mother' and navigating a career that is financially imperative as well as culturally valorized by the Black community (Barnes 2016). This places both Autumn and Dr Smith in a position where they must navigate the tensions of feeling like they cannot do enough for their child while still needing to meet financial obligations as well as cultural expectations. If you ask Dr Smith about her feelings of having to 'do it all', she simply states that 'it needs done and I haven't hit a wall yet'.

Conclusion

The focus of this chapter has been on the configuring power of a diagnostic category and its ominous potentiality for African American children, especially boys. We have called upon the notion of the syndemic to explore how an 'epidemic' of mass incarceration of Blacks (including a disproportionate number of those with mental illnesses) configures autism in ways that make it especially dangerous for young Black males. The institutional space of special education as a 'pipeline to prison' for children of colour plays a central role. The two mothers introduced in this chapter both go to enormous lengths to protect their children from the diagnosis as well as the fate of special education.

Several decades ago, the medical historian Charles Rosenberg introduced the term 'configuration' to consider how diseases are framed. He argued that 'each disease is invested with a unique configuration of social characteristics – and thus triggers disease-specific attitudinal responses. Once articulated and accepted, disease entities became "actors" in a complex social situation'. As he further noted, 'this process is deeply embedded in human history' (1989: 10). The cases we have presented here highlight the racialized figures surrounding young Black males that are so prevalent in popular imagination are systemically produced and seem virtually inescapable. It is just the case that 'autism' for children of colour is not the same disease as it is for whites. But we have not wanted simply to document another instance of the social and historical configuration of a disease category. One can hear in the indignant words of both Autumn and Dr Smith – their indigenous critiques – a keen awareness that the world could or at least *should* be different. They express moral outrage. This capacity for outrage is in itself a response that depends upon an imagined ideal of justice. A world in which their sons would be treated with equal dignity and respect, were given the same opportunities, as their white counterparts. For Dr Smith, this idealized figure, the one she aspires to create for her son, is a 'more normal'. For Autumn, in heady moments, it is the figure of a future palaeontologist. But the spectre of the prisoner, the 'gangsta', also haunts her vision.

Both of these mothers have centred much of their lives around trying to inoculate their sons against the syndemic of 'becoming nothing'. The configuring forces against which they struggle have teleological force. Everything around them seems to conspire to help produce variations of the 'nothing' that they fear. Thus, they cultivate homeplaces where they pour as much energy as they can into providing protective and nurturing environments. And yet they are also aware of the limits of what they can do. When Dr Smith says of her own capacities to provide this intensive education at night, 'I haven't hit a wall yet', she intimates that there might be a wall which she will hit sometime in the future. This is a possible future when she cannot do all that is required to keep her son 'below the radar'.

As Malcolm grew older, Autumn found it increasingly difficult to find school situations where he was not highly stigmatized, even as she was able to avoid an autism diagnosis. High school was particularly difficult for him. He was once accused of sexual harassment by a high school girl when he impulsively (as he was wont to do) went up and gave her enthusiastic hugs, and Autumn had to argue with school personnel to keep him enrolled there. Malcolm had always enjoyed physical contact. From the time he was a child, his idea of touch was an exuberant, full force connection. A hug from the young Malcolm was never delicate or tentative. If he liked you, he would throw his arms around you with a big grin. Incidents like this changed Malcolm. The last time Cheryl saw him, he was eighteen, still in high school but no longer the effervescent young man he once was. Instead, he kept his arms stiffly at his sides, unsmiling, face turned away.

Acknowledgements

Cheryl Mattingly would like to acknowledge the National Institutes of Health for grant support (HD38878) and thank her long-term collaborators Mary Lawlor and Lanita Jacobs, as well as the many researchers who have worked with her through the years. Cheryl would also like to gratefully acknowledge funding from a John Simon Guggenheim fellowship that supported some of this writing. Cheryl and Stephanie offer heartfelt thanks to Lotte Meinert for her comments on earlier drafts of this chapter. Several anonymous reviewers provided additional helpful comments. One, in particular, pointed us towards the implications of our work on the original concept of syndemic. Matthew McCoy gave some invaluable assistance in the final preparations of the chapter.

Stephanie Keeney Parks would like to thank the Parks family and all of the Black families who have allowed her into their worlds. She would also like to thank Linda Garro, Doug Hollan, H.

Samy Alim and Cheryl for their care and support throughout her graduate career.

Cheryl Mattingly
Professor, Department of Anthropology
University of Southern California

Stephanie Keeney Parks
Doctoral Student, Department of Anthropology
University of California Los Angeles

Notes

1. A version of some portions of this chapter has been published previously, from a significantly different theoretical vantage point (Mattingly 2017).
2. https://nces.ed.gov/programs/raceindicators/indicator_rda.asp, accessed 9 July 2021.
3. She decided to participate in Stephanie's research as research 'subject' and not only as a clinical and academic expert.

References

Abrahams, Roger. 1963. *Deep Down in the Jungle: Negro Narrative Folklore from the Streets of Philadelphia*, revised edn. New York: Aldine Transaction.

Alim, H. Samy. 2005. 'Hearing What's Not Said and Missing What Is: Black Language in White Public Space', in S.F. Kiesling and C. Bratt Paulston (eds), *Intercultural Discourse and Communication: The Essential Readings*. Malden, MA: Blackwell, pp. 180–197.

———. 2009. 'Hip Hop Nation Language', in Alessandro Duranti (ed.), *Linguistic Anthropology: A Reader*, 2nd edn. Malden, MA: Blackwell, pp. 272–89.

Alim, H. Samy, Geneva Smitherman and Michael Eric Dyson. 2012. *Articulate While Black: Barack Obama, Language, and Race in the US*. Oxford: Oxford University Press.

American Civil Liberties Union. 2014. 'School-to-Prison Pipeline | American Civil Liberties Union'. Retrieved 13 January 2021 from https://www.aclu.org/issues/juvenile-justice/school-prison-pipeline?redirect=fact-sheet/what-school-prison-pipeline.

Banks, Joy. 2014. 'Barriers and Supports to Postsecondary Transition: Case Studies of African American Students with Disabilities', *Remedial and Special Education* 35(1): 28–39.

Barnes, Riché J. Daniel. 2016. *Raising the Race: Black Career Women Redefine Marriage, Motherhood, and Community*. New Brunswick, NJ: Rutgers University Press.
Baugh, J. 2003. 'Linguistic Profiling', in A. Ball et al. (eds), *Black Linguistics: Language, Society, and Politics in Africa and the Americas*. London: Routledge, pp. 155–63.
Bettelheim, B. 1972. *The Empty Fortress: Infantile Autism and the Birth of the Self*. New York: Simon and Schuster.
Bucholtz, M. 2012. 'Word Up: Social Meanings of Slang in California Youth Culture', in Leila Monaghan, Jane E. Goodman and Jennifer Meta Robinson (eds), *A Cultural Approach to Interpersonal Communication* 2nd edn. Malden: Wiley-Blackwell, pp. 274–97.
Derrida, Jacques. 1994. *Specters of Marx*. New York: Routledge.
Dutta, A., C. Scguri-Geist and M. Kundu. 2009. 'Coordinator of Postsecondary Transition Services for Students with Disability', *Journal of Rehabilitation* 75(1): 10–17.
Erevelles, N. 2014. 'Crippin' Jim Crow: Disability, Dis-Location, and the School-to-Prison Pipeline', in L. Ben-Moshe, C. Chapman and A. Carey (eds), *Disability Incarcerated: Imprisonment and Disability in the United States and Canada*. London: Palgrave Macmillan, pp. 81–119.
Erickson, W., C. Lee and S. von Schrader. 2017. *Disability Statistics from the American Community Survey (ACS)*. Ithaca, NY: Cornell University Yang-Tan Institute (YTI). Retrieved 13 January 2021 from the Cornell University Disability Statistics website, www.disabilitystatistics.org.
Farmer, P. 2009. 'On Suffering and Structural Violence: A View from Below', *Race/Ethnicity: Multidisciplinary Global Contexts* 3: 11–28.
Farmer, P., et al. 2004. 'An Anthropology of Structural Violence', *Current Anthropology* 45: 305–25.
Good, Byron J. 2012. 'Phenomenology, Psychoanalysis, and Subjectivity in Java', *Ethos* 40(1): 24–36.
———. 2019. 'Hauntology: Theorizing the Spectral in Psychological Anthropology', *Ethos* 47(4): 411–26.
Gordon, Avery. 2008. *Ghostly Matters: Haunting and the Sociological Imagination*, New University of Minnesota Press edn. Minneapolis: University of Minnesota Press.
Grinker, R.R. 2007. *Unstrange Minds: Remapping the World of Autism*. New York: Basic Books.
Grinker, R.R., M. Yeargin-Allsopp and C. Boyle. 2011. 'Culture and Autism Spectrum Disorders: The Impact on Prevalence and Recognition', in D.G. Amaral, G. Dawson and D.H. Geschwind (eds), *Autism Spectrum Disorders*. New York: Oxford University Press, pp. 112–36.
Hacking, I. 1999. *The Social Construction of What?* Cambridge, MA: Harvard University Press.
Harness Goodwin, Marjorie, and H. Samy Alim. 2010. '"Whatever (Neck Roll, Eye Roll, Teeth Suck)": The Situated Coproduction of Social Categories

and Identities through Stancetaking and Transmodal Stylization', *Journal of Linguistic Anthropology* 20(1): 179–94.

Hartman, Saidiya V. 1997. *Scenes of Subjection: Terror, Slavery, and Self-Making in Nineteenth-Century America*. New York: Oxford University Press.

Hendricks, D. 2010. 'Employment and Adults with Autism Spectrum Disorders: Challenges and Strategies for Success', *Journal of Vocational Rehabilitation* 32(2): 125–34.

Hill, Jane. 2009. 'Language, Race, and White Public Space', in Alessandro Duranti (ed.), *Linguistic Anthropology: A Reader*, 2nd edn. Malden, MA: Blackwell, pp. 479–93.

Hollan, D. 2019. 'Who Is Haunted by Whom? Steps to an Ecology of Haunting', *Ethos* 47:
451–464.

hooks, bell. 1990. *Yearning: Race, Gender, and Cultural Politics*. New York: Routledge.

Hurlbutt, K., and L. Chalmers. 2004. 'Employment and Adults with Asperger Syndrome', *Focus on Autism and Other Developmental Disabilities* 19(4): 215–22.

Kanner, L. 1949. 'Problems of Nosology and Psychodynamics of Early Infantile Autism', *American Journal of Orthopsychiatry* 19: 416–26.

King, M.D., and P.S. Bearman. 2011. 'Socioeconomic Status and the Increased Prevalence of Autism in California', *American Sociological Review* 76: 320–46.

Kochman, Thomas. 1969. '"Rapping" in the Black Ghetto', *Trans-Action* 6: 26–34.

Kogan, M.D., et al. 2009. 'Prevalence of Parent-Reported Diagnosis of Autism Spectrum Disorder among Children in the US', *Pediatrics* 124: 1395–403.

Lincoln, Martha, and Bruce Lincoln. 2015. 'Toward a Critical Hauntology: Bare Afterlife and the Ghosts of Ba Chúc', *Comparative Studies in Society and History* 57(1): 191–220.

Liu, K.Y., M. King and P.S. Bearman. 2010. 'Social Influence and the Autism Epidemic', *American Journal of Sociology* 115: 1387–434.

Losen, D.J. 2018. 'Disabling Punishment: The Need for Remedies to the Disparate Loss of Instruction Experienced by Black Students with Disabilities'. Retrieved 13 January 2021 from the Center for Civil Rights Remedies at the Civil Rights Project website, https://today.law.harvard.edu/wp-content/uploads/2018/04/disabling-punishment-report-.pdf.

Louw, Maria. 2018. 'Haunting as Moral Engine: Ethical Striving and Moral Aporias among Sufis in Uzbekistan', in Cheryl Mattingly, Rasmus Dyring, Maria Louw and Thomas Schwarz Wentzer (eds), *Moral Engines: Exploring the Ethical Drives in Human Life*. New York: Berghahn, pp. 83–99.

Mandell, D., et al. 2002. 'Race Differences in the Age at Diagnosis among Medicaid-Eligible Children with Autism', *Journal of the American Academy of Child and Adolescent Psychiatry* 41 (December): 1447–53.

Mandell, D., et al. 2007. 'Disparities in Diagnoses Received Prior to a Diagnosis of Autism Spectrum Disorder', *Journal of Autism and Developmental Disorders* 37: 1795–802.

Mandell, D., et al. 2009. 'Racial/Ethnic Disparities in the Identification of Children with Autism Spectrum Disorders', *American Journal of Public Health* 99: 493–98.

Mattingly, C. 2010. *The Paradox of Hope: Journeys through a Clinical Borderland.* Berkeley: University of California Press.

Mattingly, C. 2017. 'Autism and the Ethics of Care: A Phenomenological Investigation into the Contagion of Nothing', Special Issue, 'Social Contagion and Cultural Epidemics', L. Gron and L. Meinert (eds), *Ethos* 45(2): 250–70.

McDermott, R.P. 1993. 'The Acquisition of a Child by a Learning Disability', in S. Chaiklin and J. Lave (eds), *Understanding Practice: Perspectives on Activity and Context.* Cambridge: Cambridge University Press, pp. 269–304.

Merikangas, K.R., et al. 2010. 'Lifetime Prevalence of Mental Disorders in US Adolescents: Results from the National Comorbidity Study-Adolescent Supplement' (Ncs-a), *Journal of the American Academy of Child and Adolescent Psychiatry* 49: 980.

Mitchell-Kernan, Claudia. 1971. *Language Behavior in a Black Urban Community.* University of California, Berkeley: Language Behavior Research Laboratory.

——— . 1972. 'Signifying and Marking: Two Afro-American Speech Acts', in John J. Gumperz and Dell Hymes (eds), *Directions in Sociolinguistics.* New York: Holt, Rinehart and Winston, pp. 161–79.

Morgan, Marcyliena. 1994. 'The African American Speech Community: Reality and Sociolinguistics', in *Language and the Social Construction of Identity in Creole Situations.* Los Angeles: CAAS Publications, pp. 121–48.

Morrison, Toni. 1987. *Beloved: A Novel.* New York: Knopf.

National Association for the Advancement of Colored People (NAACP). N.d.a. 'Criminal Justice Fact Sheet'. Retrieved 13 January 2021 from https://naacp.org/resources/criminal-justice-fact-sheet.

Nguyen, V.K., and K. Peschard. 2003. 'Anthropology, Inequality, and Disease: A Review', *Annual Review of Anthropology* 32: 447–74.

Noguera, P.A. 2003. 'The Trouble with Black Boys: The Role and Influence of Environmental and Cultural Factors on the Academic Performance of African American Males', *Urban Education* 38(4): 431–59.

Ochs, E., and O. Solomon. 2010. 'Autistic Sociality', *Ethos: Journal of the Society for Psychological Anthropology* 38(1): 69–92.

Overton, T., C. Fielding and R. de Alba. 2007. 'Differential Diagnosis of Hispanic Children Referred for Autism Spectrum Disorders: Complex Issues', *Journal of Autism and Developmental Disorders* 37: 1996–2007.

Pew Research Center. 2013. 'King's Dream Remains an Elusive Goal; Many Americans See Racial Disparities', Pew Research Center's Social and Demographic Trends Project. Retrieved from https://www.pewsocialtrends.

org/2013/08/22/kings-dream-remains-an-elusive-goal-many-americans-see-racial-disparities/.
Powell, Tunette, and S. Keeney Parks. Forthcoming. 'They Never Listen to the Parent: Parent Narratives at the Intersection of Racism, Education, and Disability', in D. Hines, M. Boveda and E.J. Lindo (eds), *Racism by Another Name: Black Students, Overrepresentation, and the Carceral State of Special Education*. Greenwich, CT: Information Age Publishing.
Rapp, Rayna. 2011. 'A Child Surrounds this Brain: The Future of Neurological Difference
According to Scientists, Parents and Diagnosed Young Adults', M. Pickersgill and I. Van Keulen (eds), *Sociological Reflections on the Neurosciences (Advances in Medical Sociology, Vol. 13)*, Bingley: Emerald Group Publishing Limited, pp. 3–26.
Robertson, S.M. 2010. 'Neurodiversity, Quality of Life, and Autistic Adults: Shifting Research and Professional Focuses onto Real-Life Challenges', *Disability Studies Quarterly* 30(1): 27.
Rosenberg, C. 1989. 'Disease in History: Frames and Framers. Framing Disease: The Creation and Negotiation of Explanatory Schemes', *The Milbank Quarterly* 67 (Supplement 1): 1–15.
Salamon, Gayle. 2018. *The Life and Death of Latisha King: A Critical Phenomenology of Transphobia*. New York: New York University Press.
Seeberg, J., and L. Meinert. 2015. 'Can Epidemics Be Noncommunicable? Reflections on the Spread of Noncommunicable Diseases', *Medicine Anthropology Theory* 2(2): 54–71.
Sharpe, Christina. 2016. *In the Wake: On Blackness and Being*. Durham, NC: Duke University Press.
Shattuck, P.T., et al. 2012. 'Postsecondary Education and Employment among Youth with an Autism Spectrum Disorder', *Pediatrics* 129: 1042–49.
Silverman, C. 2008. 'Brains, Pedigrees, and Promises: Lessons from the Politics of Autism Genetics', in S. Gibbons and C. Novas (eds), *Biosocialities, Genetics and the Social Sciences: Making Biologies and Identities*. New York: Routledge, pp. 38–55.
———. 2012. *Understanding Autism: Parents, Doctors, and the History of a Disorder*. Princeton, NJ: Princeton University Press.
Singer, Merrill, et al. 2017. 'Syndemics and the Biosocial Conception of Health', *Lancet* 389(10072): 941–50.
Smitherman, Geneva. 1973. 'The Power of the Rap: The Black Idiom and the New Black Poetry', *Twentieth Century Literature: A Scholarly and Critical Journal* 19: 259–74.
———. 1977. *Talkin and Testifyin: The Language of Black America*. Detroit: Wayne State University Press.
———. 1999. *Talkin That Talk: Language, Culture and Education in African America*. New York: Routledge.
———. 2000. *Black Talk: Words and Phrases from the Hood to the Amen Corner*, rev. edn. Boston, MA: Mariner Books.

Spillers, Hortense. 2003. *Black, White and in Color*. Chicago: University of Chicago Press.
Taylor, J.L., and M.M. Seltzer. 2011. 'Employment and Post-Secondary Educational Activities for Young Adults with Autism Spectrum Disorders during the Transition to Adulthood', *Journal of Autism and Developmental Disorders* 41(5): 566–74.
Thomas, Jamie, and Susan Nix. 2017. 'Use of Social Narratives as an Evidence-Based Practice to Support Employment of Young Adults with Autism Spectrum Disorders: A Practitioner's Guide', *Journal of the American Academy of Special Education Professionals* (Winter): 163–69.
Wald, J., and D.J. Losen. 2003. 'Defining and Redirecting a School-to-Prison Pipeline', *New Directions for Youth Development* 99: 9–15.

Chapter 4
Configuring Affection
Family Experiences of Obesity and Social Contagion in Denmark

Lone Grøn

Karsten: Well, if anything is contagious, I think it is commercials in the television. Advertisements for that which has easily accessible calories that sticks to your bones. Those are the most widespread. So ... I think that for me is contagion.

Heidi: I think you hear messages from the media and so on: 'Eat healthy!', 'Lose weight!' And then, if you think: 'Now I will go grocery shopping, it has to be healthy, it has to varied, it has to be good' – but then it is super expensive. So there is a mixed message in the prices, I mean, the cost of buying it. If you are pressured financially then unhealthy is the cheapest.

Bettina: Well, I would say being busy. We are too busy. We do not have time for each other, we do not have time for presence, we do not have time for being in the present. It is contagious by there being no space for getting out the innermost emotions. There is no space to stand there on your feet knowing 'Who am I, deep down'? Because we do not have time for that! Yes, to fill this emotional gap, then I think, well, we get the chemistry by eating something, which tastes good. This is where it comes – whether it is chocolate or McDonald's or milkshake – or whatever it is called.

Over the last decades, obesity has come to occupy both popular and health-related political imaginations, and media headlines have declared the emergence of an obesity epidemic. This raises the question of whether you can talk about contagion in lifestyle-related epidemics (Seeberg and Meinert 2015), that is, social contagion rather than biological infection. If so, how does obesity spread and social contagion happen? Are television commercials contagious, as Karsten explains, at least those for the 'calories that stick to your bones'? Or is it, as Heidi points out, the difference in price between healthy and unhealthy food items that leads to more people becoming obese? Or do life stresses, as claimed by Bettina, and lack of time to be present with your innermost emotions create a susceptibility to obesity? Lack of time, in other words, to meet the world through resonance (Rosa 2019).

For several decades now, social science researchers have voiced critiques of the way obesity tends to be understood mainly in terms of individual lifestyle. The input/output model of obesity, which

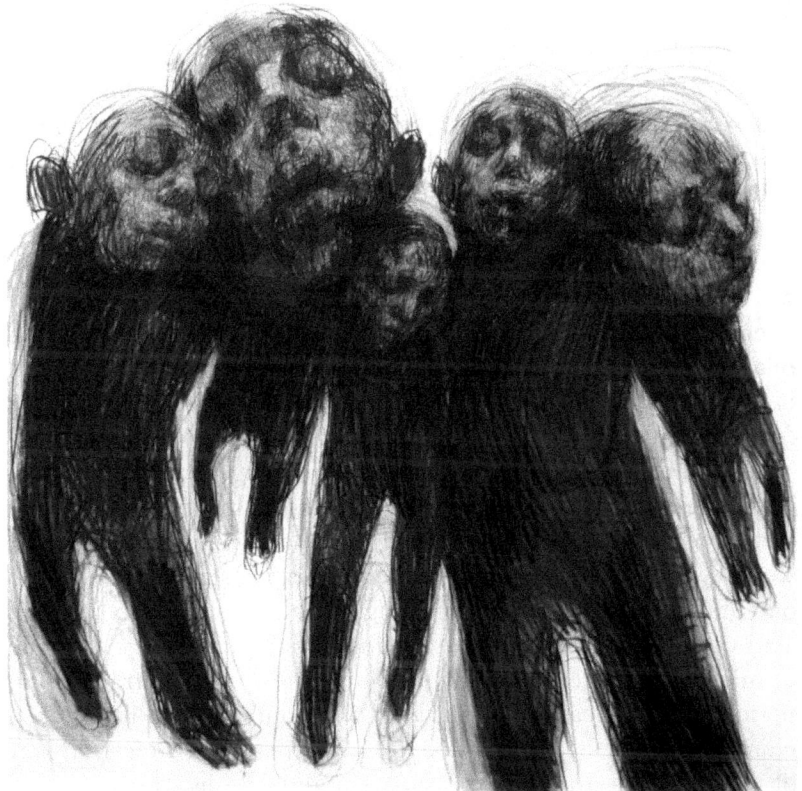

Figure 4.1. 'Conviction 6' by Maria Speyer. Photo by and courtesy of Maria Speyer, www.mariaspeyer.com.

posits that weight gain and loss can be explained as a matter of energy intake and expenditure, has been criticized for reducing the complexities and unresolved questions surrounding the obesity epidemic (see e.g. Gard and Wright 2005; McCullough and Hardin 2013; Wright and Harwood 2009). Specifically, critiques have been raised against individualizing a phenomenon that has strong social, structural and historical underpinnings, thereby stigmatizing people who are overweight or obese, and contributing to the negative effects of living with obesity (Boero 2007; Greenhalgh 2015; Moffat 2010), suggesting instead notions of social networks (Christakis and Fowler 2007), the obesogenic society (Swinburn et al. 2011), fat metabolism and insecurity (Sørensen 2014) and metabolic living (Solomon 2016). These critiques, thus, lend some credibility to the multitude of co-existing causal pathways indicated by the above quotes from Heidi, Karsten and Bettina.

In fieldwork from 2001–03, 2013–14 and ongoing, I have approached obesity through the experiences of Danish families in which obesity has run across generations. Even though families know obesity intimately, uncertainties and doubts prevail, about specific causes and their relationships to other causes, as well as what to do about it. This has prompted me to suggest the notion of affection as a phenomenological theory of social contagion (Grøn 2017a). I have taken my main inspiration from the responsive phenomenology of Bernhard Waldenfels,[1] which posits a dynamic relationship between the call of the alien (in German *das Fremde*, i.e. alienness) in our experience and our responses to such calls.

The alien call highlights the pathic or suffering side of experience, while the responses capture the more agentive dimensions. Waldenfels characterizes the pathic side of this dynamic by the notion of af-fect, separating the prefix in order to highlight that when we are affected by the alien, it is by something outside our grasp, our own order of things (Waldenfels 2011: 26–27). The notion of affection, thus, points to contagion in the mode of uncertainty (Stevenson 2014; Whyte 1997). In contrast to the notion of biological infection, affection connotes two interlinked characteristics: the profound *intersubjectivity* and *indeterminacy* of causal pathways (Grøn 2017a). The drawing by Maria Speyer[2] illustrates how, in lived experience, it becomes difficult to know where one person ends and another begins, and how we are

Configuring Affection

differentially affected by that which befalls us. Thus, the notion of affection challenges both the idea of individual lifestyle in contemporary debates and interventions targeting obesity *and* the linear and demarcated causal pathways that characterize epidemiological approaches to obesity. It presents, instead, an experience-near and anthropological approach that takes seriously the idea that academically demarcated territories between disciplines, and between individuals, others and the world, might not be helpful for understanding how obesity spreads.

In this chapter, I focus on the configuration of diverse biosocial affections in the obesity epidemic through an exploration of family drawings or maps of relatedness, which – like Maria Speyer's drawing – demonstrate a profound intersubjectivity and indeterminacy in the lived experience of social contagion. Taking up Meinert and Seeberg's suggestion in their Introduction to this volume that the notion of configuration can create a framework for describing the figures and con-figures that create epidemic processes of contagion, I will add two further characteristics to the notion of affection.

1. Family experiences of contagion highlight affection as mutuality and mattering, as love and belonging. Family affection, however, is both nourishing and poisonous, which makes contagion as affection especially haunting (Meinert and Grøn 2019). You cannot do without it, it nourishes you, but it also hurts you. Furthermore, the affective ties do not adhere to distinctions between what is biological and what is social but emerge between material, biological, psychological, cultural, social and historical processes. Affective ties emerge not only between people, but between people, things and the world (Kuan forthcoming; Stewart 2007). As demonstrated within affect theory, affect can be seen as a moving, transpersonal force or energy that compels, attracts and provokes (Rutherford 2016) between the most intimate and the most impersonal domains (ibid.; Mazzarella 2017). Social inequality, lifestyles, Danish 'hygge', genes, family love and trauma intersect in the configuring of affection.
2. The configuration of diverse affections is specific and particular, and we must take an interest in the particular times and places, and in the particular and situated family situations

and histories. This allows us to distinguish between different kinds of intergenerational and societal transmission, which lead to different kinds of obesity, not only between families but also within them. Obesity thus appears not as a monolithic category, but as obesities in the plural.

One further inspiration for my exploration of family affection in the obesity epidemic are kinship studies that aspire to take us beyond the biology–culture dichotomy (Bamford and Leach 2009; Carsten 2004; Franklin and McKinnon 2001; Sahlins 2013; Schneider 1980) and offer glimpses of how the world might look 'through "non-genealogical" eyes'[3] (Bamford and Leach 2009: 19). Here Viveiros de Castro's contribution regarding the Amazonian kinship model serves as an excellent example. He reveals a world of analogous kinship flows (Wagner 1977) where yams can be our lineage brothers, or where jaguars reveal themselves as our cannibal brothers-in-law (Viveiros de Castro 2009: 249). Finally, we can also think of family affection through the notion of heritage, more specifically pre-genetic and pre-medical notions of heritage (Müller-Wille and Rheinberger 2007) where heredity was both more than and different from the scientific discipline of genetics (ibid.: 13) and where heredity and environment – or nature and nurture – were not seen as opposites (ibid.: 3). In such an understanding of heredity, place, historical time, belongings, relations and bodies might all play important roles in how things run in families. Here Angela Garcia's work on inheritance as 'querencia' points to how heroin addiction can be linked to soil, to property, to kinship, to blood, to love – and to structural and economic developments over time (Garcia 2014).

The Family and Relatedness Maps

I have known the families in this chapter for two decades.[4] The data used for this chapter stem from my second period of fieldwork (2013–14), when I explored family experiences of the spread of obesity. Methodologically, I relied on drawings that the families made of how obesity ran in their families and extended social networks.

I did not ask for the maps to be drawn in specific ways, but asked the drawer(s) to include those that mattered most, whether they be kin, friends or colleagues (or, as we see in one of the drawings, power animals and angels), and start wherever they wanted on a large piece of paper. Two drawings were made by one person, one by a couple, and one by a family of five. There are obvious differences between the ways these drawings portray a network. The individual drawings portray the network as experienced from the perspective of the drawer. Those by the couple and the family are co-creations, in which the process of drawing itself tends to highlight family dynamics.

Initially, the drawings were intended as a way to pay systemic attention to kinship and relatedness in the obesity epidemic, and even more specifically to map those who were or had been obese in the family and broader relatedness network. But the drawings – and the process of drawing – turned out to be about so much more. The initial drawing of the sometimes quite large relatedness network took several hours and prompted stories of family conflicts, passions, hurts and strivings over time, many of which I had not heard about in the extended time period I had known these families. Only at the end did we get to mark and discuss the distribution and spread of obesity.

Rita's Drawing

Rita places her main people as interlinked hearts at the centre of the drawing: her mother, father, brother, herself, her grandmother on her mother's side, and her four children are drawn into this heart formation. She then divides the paper into four big subsections: upper left 'family', upper right 'friends' she shares with her husband, lower left 'friends' that are her own, and lower right 'work' relations. Finally, she adds a section to the right of the central heart formation named 'personal helpers', which are angels and power animals (eagle, bear, unicorn and wolf).

The stars, which mark obesity, are clustered in the family sections of the drawing, which together with the hearts set the affective tone of family contagion – big hearts and big people. Rita marks her father, mother, brother, brother's children and wife, her own husband and two elder daughters as well as her favourite cousin, four of her husband's five siblings and two of their spouses as obese. Three of her friends and a spouse of a friend are also marked with a star. In subsequent interviews, Rita and her family went into extensive

Lone Grøn

discussions on how obesity spreads, mentioning Danish *hygge* (see Karsten's formulations in the next section), McDonald's restaurants and fast food more generally. And – as we saw in the quote from Bettina, the eldest daughter in this family, at the beginning of this chapter – the stress and loneliness of modern life, where too much attention is given to numbers, measures and effectivity in all areas of life.

However, in the course of the drawing Rita talks about the causes of obesity in more intimate and relational ways. Over the two decades I have known her, she has repeatedly mentioned her mother when asked about causes of her own overweight. The contents of these talks have changed, from how she felt her mother did not approve of her husband or of one or more of her children at different points in time, to more opaque statements of not knowing how, but just that 'it' had to do with her mother.[5] In this drawing session, she talks about a lack of self-worth:

> My lovely mother has an amazingly low sense of self-worth without having any ground for it. She is so competent. She has kept the home perfectly, she has raised my brother and me, she has sewn all her own clothes, and she has always been an amazing cook. And everything she takes on she does so well, knitting and ... she can do everything! But

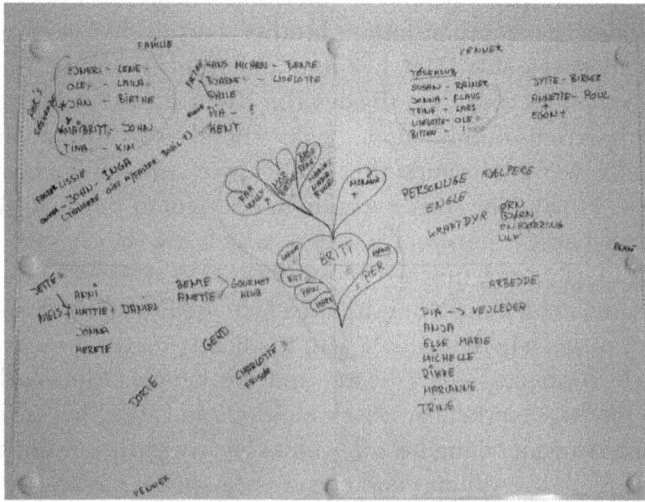

Figure 4.2. Rita's drawing of her family and friend network. Persons marked with stars are considered obese by Rita. Photo by Tove Nyholm.

she never had a proper sense of self-worth. She is born number two, no, number one. But then, the next was a boy and a boy had more worth.

Here she explains more about her uncle, who actually had a very hard life. He was an alcoholic and committed suicide. She then recounts a childhood memory:

> I remember one time – and I was not very old and I often went driving with my mother and father. I loved coming along, my mother loved coming along, and then we just sat in the car. ... Well, then one time when we were driving and I was sitting between them, then I thought, 'I will never be as competent and good as them'. No, now I am crying. Oh God [silence] I was not more than five, I think. How can you define that when you are five?

Her reflections on her mother's and her own sense of self-worth are not specific to obesity but include work life and what they dared to wish for in life, but when I ask her if her obesity can be linked to anybody in the map, she immediately again points to her mother. However, in this talk she also conveys a very different form of affection. When I ask Rita what her husband would say about his overweight, she responds:

> He says that it is because he likes food, he says it is dangerous to have a wife that cooks so well! And he says, that I am overweight because I had four children. So he takes part of the blame. He says: 'It's my fault'.

I reply that his explanations seem more hands-on and light-hearted than hers and she agrees. In fact, she does not disagree with her husband's explanation. Rather, the liking of food, the preference for boys over girls, the danger of having a good cook for a wife, the four pregnancies and the mother's gift to her of a low sense of self-worth co-exist and coalesce. It does seem, though, that there is a gendered configuration at play here, where female bodies and modes of care and belonging are more contagious and come with an added weight, whether through cooking, pregnancies (for which her husband does take part of the blame) or mother–daughter transmissions.

The lived experience of contagion that we see here does not emerge as a causal relation between demarcated units in a linear fashion but as affection characterized by profound intersubjectivity and indeterminacy. Rita knows and remembers clearly how her mother always believed in her. How, then, did her mother's low self-worth (for which there were no obvious grounds besides being born a girl) settle into a five-year-old (also a girl) in a car seat? And, as she says, how can you even define that when you are five?

In affection it is hard to determine where one person stops and another begins (Grøn 2017a), and from the child's perspective it might not make sense to speak of contagion as something imposed from the outside and handed across a relation (Han and Brandel 2019). Rather, this is a form of life in which the child is completely immersed, where there is no sedimented concept of 'father' and 'mother', 'son' or 'sister' (ibid.). An affective environment in which glances, moods, movements, silences and sounds of kin constitute 'the sub-social', a level of family life which is hard to grasp and document, but where contagious connections often happen (Kuan 2019). Such modes of affection are profoundly intersubjective, also in the sense that intersubjectivity constitutes the environment, the content and the pathway of the contagious connections (Meinert and Grøn 2019).

The Couples' Drawing

The next drawing is done by a couple, Karsten and Tina. The drawing happens in phases. First, they co-draw their core family as the central unit: Karsten, Tina and their only daughter. Then he draws his side of the family, and finally Tina draws hers. They mark obesity by a thick black line and it becomes clear that obesity runs in his family, not in hers.

Elsewhere, I have relied on Karsten's poetic and competent renderings of Danish *hygge*, that is, a both traditional and still valued form of socializing through (often excessive) eating and drinking as one prominent site where affection happens (Grøn 2017a):

> Karsten: Well, in my family we have always appreciated ... we could sit around the table for hours, you know. And enjoy the food. And enjoy the company ... and the atmosphere there, the music, the wine, and all of this that just flows, right?
> Lone: Uh huh. So you couldn't just sit around the table ... you couldn't get the same out of it, if there was no food and wine on the table?
> Karsten: No. No. I could not imagine ... we have had these gathering of cousins and they have been like the event of the year ... where we

have got everyone together for some good food, you know. Then you have a good talk with your cousins: 'How's it going', 'How are you', and that kind of thing, you know. And it is not like, you know, there's not one quiet moment. On the contrary, you can hear ... we have some recordings from a cell phone, where the atmosphere [making a rising movement with his hand]...

Lone: ... rises and rises, ha-ha!

Karsten: Suddenly they say that the music has to be turned up! Then people just shout a bit louder [Karsten shouts out loud sounding like a trumpet, to demonstrate how the volume of the conversation increases]. And, if they had been bored it would have been just like [making now a falling gesture with his hand], you know. And that ... no, no.

Lone: No ... so there is a connection between food and alcohol and togetherness?

Karsten: Yes! I would say that, good food, well I think what characterises my side of the family is that if there's good food on the table then the atmosphere will immediately be up there in the red zone! (Grøn 2017a: 189)

Here, affection happens, in Karsten's words, through the 'inhalation' of food, drink and company, an affective integration of

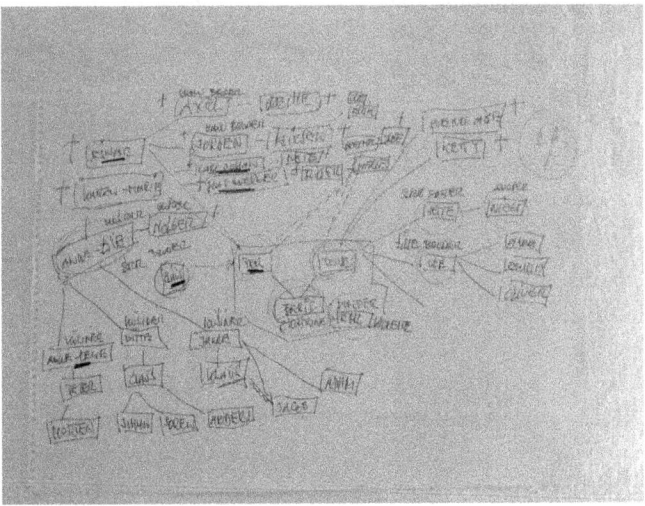

Figure 4.3. Karsten and Tina's drawing of their family and friend network. Persons underlined are considered obese by Karsten and Tina. Photo by Tove Nyholm.

others and things into one's own body, a merging of self and other 'in the red zone'. According to Karsten's poetic formulation, being in the red zone represents the highest possible 'form of beauty', but also, unfortunately, this is a site where affection of obesity happens (ibid.). However, in this drawing session it becomes adamantly clear that while *hygge* is a cherished practice in both families, only in Karsten's family does this lead to some family members becoming overweight. But when I ask Karsten about people in the drawing whom he relates to his obesity, he points – among others – to Tina's mother:

> Karsten: Well I used to say that the cause of my gaining weight was Tina's mother, because she cooked so well. I have had a hard time saying no, many times. When you came to Western Jutland and to Tina's mother ... the food was always tip-top!
> Tina: Yes and gravy wasn't too bad, either.
> Karsten: I remember, the gravy! Those 'shitty eggs' we got served out there, I loved that milk sauce and eggs and the mustard. And at Christmas, your mother was the earth champion, the world champion, in making *ris a la mande* and pork roast. She even put sugar in the red cabbage. I got that too, it tasted damn good!
> Lone: So even though we might think this is unhealthy, it sounds like it was fantastic. I mean, what she could do, and not only for Karsten...
> Tina: Also for everybody else, yes.
> Karsten: We all enjoyed it out there. Even doggy who – semi fat dog, it was so big you had to carry it up the stairs, right.
> Tina: But, ah ... Well, actually there are no overweight people in my family. We haven't, you know, gained weight.

We see in this conversational drawing between Karsten and Tina how that which is a cause of obesity is also a cause of happiness, joy, care and love for both of them, for the entire family. The nourishing and the poisonous co-exist in the gravy, the 'shitty eggs', the red cabbage – and in kinship affection (Meinert and Grøn 2019). And as in the previous example there are strong gendered differences in the configuration of affection. Rita immediately points to her mother when asked about relational causes of obesity, even though her father was in fact more obese, and both Rita's husband and Karsten ascribe their obesity to exposure to women who cook too well, demonstrating the ambiguous yet gendered pathways of family affection.

While Tina and Karsten share the joys of mutually recollecting her mother's excellent cooking, in the following part of the conversation they part ways: Tina is adamant that Karsten should lose weight, he is diabetic, he has heart and back problems. She does not want to lose him, she says, both she and their daughter worry about him. Karsten on his side explains that he asked the doctor if he would become happy if he lost weight. The doctor responded that he would become thinner; happy he did not know. For Karsten the regime that comes with weight loss robs him of that which gives life its value: not only the enjoyment of good food, but the enjoyment of good food in the good company of others. Danish *hygge*, or the highest 'form of beauty'.

This is corroborated by how Karsten talks about his brother who is also obese – and lives alone. Karsten finds his stacks of pizza and ready-made food boxes appalling. I ask Karsten if he is on his brother's back just the way Tina is on his. Karsten agrees and Tina adds: 'Yes, and my sister is too!' Karsten: 'My daughter is on my back, too! The only one who stays neutral is my friend Paul. His wife we just ask to keep quiet! Because she is chubby herself!' Tina laughs: 'She is not – stop!' They both break into laughter.

Summing up, not only obesity but also joy, conflicts and care around obesity and weight loss run in the family, as we will see in the last two family drawings.

Susanne's Drawing

Susanne starts by placing herself at the centre of the empty paper and then builds up the network from there. Each person appears as one part in a cluster or organism of multiple parts. As we talk, dramas, conflicts and alliances between family members, ex-family members, friends and colleagues unfold and it becomes quite clear that Susanne occupies the position of one who cares – even for those she does not particularly like, or who have 'left' the family through divorce. Through the process of drawing, she becomes quite overwhelmed and states that perhaps all this caretaking is why she gets so exhausted.

Specifically in relation to obesity, Susanne draws a circle around the people – family, friends and colleagues – who are or have been obese. While there are some overweight people in all categories, there is a marked clustering around kin relations. However, there are different kinds of obesity. Susanne explains:

> Susanne: Well, there is a difference because they [she points to her mother and maternal aunt] were overweight, while my grandmother and her sister, I mean, that was extreme. A little bit as I used to be. When I was a kid, when my grandmother's sister died, I don't know if it was just something they said, but they said that she was so big, they couldn't fit her into the coffin. Like, they had to puncture something. Maybe it was just something they made up, but still it was like, when she sat in the couch, her stomach touched the floor! So, you can say you can be overweight where it is still a little shapely. That wasn't the case with her. And my grandmother was also very, very large.
> Lone: So this was in the 1960s, right?
> Susanne: Yes, I was born in 1962 so in the 1960s. And, my mother was overweight, but not like, not that way, extreme. She also had a sister who was overweight, but she was like a beanstalk as a child. When my mother had children, she got really big.
> Lone: So they were both overweight, but in different ways?
> Susanne: Yes, but they didn't have the same father. My mother was still a little overweight after having us three girls, but she lost a lot of weight, when she went on the pill. The doctors have told me that they think

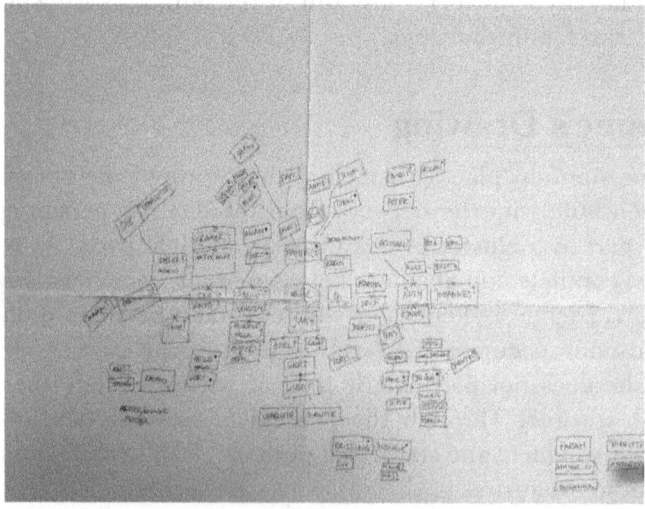

Figure 4.4. Susanne's drawing of her family and friend network. Persons marked with circles (red in the original drawing) are considered obese by Susanne. Photo by Tove Nyholm.

Configuring Affection

there was something in the birth control pills my mother took. This was in '67, something was in them that made her lose weight, and that is why they think that I also lacked something. Because in my puberty, not only did I get overweight, but I just stopped growing. You know, my hands are small, I've got small feet, and I'm not very tall. They say that today they would have looked into it more. Maybe I should have been given growth hormones, because both my sisters are normal height and have normal-sized feet and so on. And they have been able to lose weight in the normal way, which I never could.

Lone: So they are more like the same body type? But you have the same genes, don't you?

Susanne: Yes. Well, it's probably also – apart from there being something genetic – then I think it's about how we were raised on potatoes and gravy, right? And we weren't raised to do sports. There was no money for that. You know, we were, I was a grown up before I was introduced to salads. It was my grandmother who introduced us to it, that you could eat raw vegetables. (Grøn 2020: 10)

While obesity has run in this family for generations, it does so in different ways. Obesities in the plural run in this family. Susanne's maternal grandmother's sister was so obese that they could not fit her into her coffin, or at least so she was told as a child. Her mother and aunt were overweight, but less extremely so, and while her aunt was slim as a child, her mother lost weight when she started taking birth control pills. Something was in the pills that might have made it impossible for Susanne to lose weight through dieting, which her sisters have been able to do. This shows that obesity is not one 'thing', not a monolithic category. Even though you are from the same family and share the same parental genes, one person's obesity can be constituted by different affective configurations than another's.

Furthermore, it is not all about genetic disposition and chemical substances – there is more to this picture. The family was very poor, there was no money for sports, and Susanne was grown up before she learned that you could eat raw vegetables. As Heidi, Rita's second daughter, remarked in the opening quotes of this chapter, there is a mixed message in the discrepancy between national health advice and the prices of food items: 'If you are pressured financially, then unhealthy is the cheapest'. While all three sisters have done well for themselves, have mid-level educations and work in the social and care professions, during their childhoods their family was very poor and they were all bullied at school. However, even here there are slight differences in the configuration of affections. Susanne's sister, Bente, explains that the bullying did not affect Susanne in the same way as it did the two other sisters, because she was so competent in school.

What emerges from Susanne's relatedness drawing is a configuration of diverse biological, social, structural and historical phenomena within which generational and relational dynamics of sameness and difference play out (Grøn 2020). In lived experience, you cannot pinpoint exact causal chains or delineate distinct causal fields as *either* biological *or* social. Rather, we can learn how family members see and experience particular configurations in their lives and family histories – where phenomena from domains we often perceive as distinct co-exist, give rise to and feed on one another. More recent family events give further evidence of this cross-fertilization between the biological and the social.

Over the course of one year, Susanne and her two sisters have gastric bypass surgeries. They have had a lifetime of evidence that this is the only way out. Susanne's sisters might have been able to lose weight on diverse diets, but each time they have gained back what they lost, along with an added five or ten kilos. When the drawing session takes place three years have passed, and the sisters have changed remarkably. The transformation has been on many levels, not only body size. Susanne's sister, Bente, has also divorced her husband and met a new boyfriend. As she says, surgery was the last but not an easy way out.

In a remarkable way, the sisters' cutting of their intestines affects Bente's daughter Marie. After her mother and aunts have surgeries, Marie has had to carry the too many kilos on her own, and not until half a year before this drawing session does she start to lose weight. When asked why this happened, Marie repeats that she does not know, because she had tried the same weight loss strategies many times before. She then says it is a miracle and ascribes this transformation to the songs of Christoffer, a blond curly-haired and blue-eyed popstar who has teenage girls screaming at his arrival – which makes the other family members laugh. In another interview Susanne explains that Marie has changed as a person. Before, she was so dependent on her mother, and Bente adds that their relationship had to change after the surgery – they could not share meals or go shopping for oversize clothes like they used to.

We see in this family event the cutting of intestines, family bonds and practices (Grøn 2020). The transmission of obesity is not experienced as biological *or* cultural. Rather, genes and growth hormones (lacking or provided in birth control pills) intersect with being raised without sports or salads, which again intersects with poverty and social class. The family is haunted by configurations, which give rise to obesities of diverse kinds and shapes, and the sisters see no other way out than to cut.

The cutting then opens up a space for the new to emerge – a new body, a new boyfriend, a new mother–daughter relationship – but also leaves an open wound. For years, Marie carries the weight of the family and bears testimony to the nourishing *and* poisonous affections of family life. Over time, the cutting of one generation's intestines affects the next, in ways that Marie terms 'a miracle'. As we saw with Rita's and her mother's low self-esteem, such intergenerational mother–daughter affections move in mysterious ways. Marie loses weight and later meets a boyfriend – named Christoffer! Affection crosses personal and generational boundaries, as well as boundaries between the biological and the social, the virtual and the real.

The Family Drawing

This is a co-drawing by a family of five: the father Peter, the mother Mette and the children Hannah, Sussie and Stefanie. The design emerges from the co-drawing, and a concern over who gets to write whom on the paper. This is a merged family: both Mette and Peter have been married before and have several children from those marriages, as well as two shared children, Sussie and Stefanie. Mette intervenes quite often to mark certain people as 'Hannah's people', telling her: 'You can write your father into the picture' or 'this person you can draw with you' (meaning at her position in the drawing), and 'this person belongs to you, too'. Hannah is Mette's daughter from her previous marriage; she has learning difficulties and no longer lives at home. Mette seeks to make her feel as related to this network drawing as the two younger daughters, who still live at home.

Lone Grøn

They mark obesity with a circle around the person's name. Obesity is distributed among several kinds of relationships in this drawing. In Mette's and especially Peter's family, several family members of both previous and present generations, including Peter and Mette, have been overweight. But there are also several obese persons among friends,[6] neighbours and colleagues.

When it comes to the family members who are present, the circles are drawn with caution. Both Hannah and Sussie struggle with weight issues – the family debate whether they should be marked as overweight or not. They agree that Hannah should not and explain that Sussie has been quite overweight, but has lost fifteen kilos due to a longer stay at boarding school. Sussie is quite explicit in stating that her home is not conducive to weight loss. The youngest sister Stefanie, however, is slim and fit. She looks like a model, they say.

> Mette: She is a changeling. She got switched at birth…
> Hannah: Yeah, she always says: 'I am fat!' Then I say: 'Bring out a lump'.
> Sussie: Such a small one…
> Hannah: Yes. Then I say: 'Look at the rest of us! Ours is twice as big…'.
> Peter: What's the name of your lump?
> Sussie: Is it Gunnar?

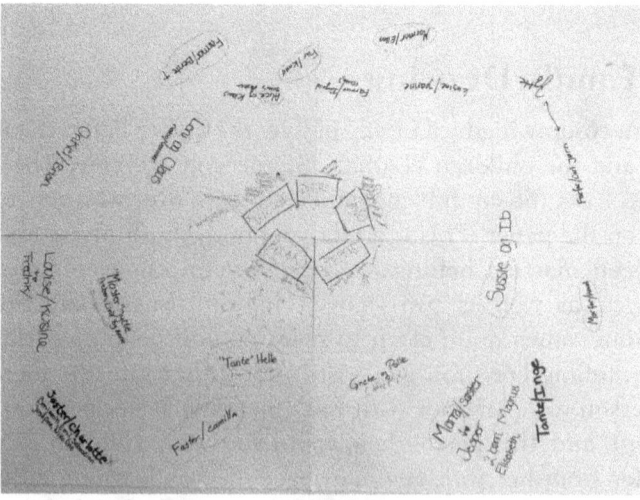

Figure 4.5. Peter, Mette, Hannah, Sussie and Stefanie's drawing of their family and friend network. Persons marked with circles (red in the original drawing) are considered obese by them. Photo by Tove Nyholm.

Stefanie: It has changed name often. I can't remember.

Sussie: Gunnar? Erik?

Lone: What do you think? They say you got switched at birth, and that they have the lumps, not you … they don't think you have a weight issue.

Stefanie: No, well, I don't think so either. But at times I do feel that I have kind of, a little…

Mette: You want a six-pack and good muscles, right?

Stefanie: Yes, but sometimes I do feel I have a little extra. And it annoys me! That you do not get it!

Mette: But a small lump can take up a lot of space.

Stefanie: Yes! It can actually!

Lone: And do the rest of you find it annoying that she is concerned about such a small lump?

Sussie: Well, if she talks about it all the time, then it is a bit like: But haven't you seen me? Right? Also, it's not very nice if we are in the bathroom where we like to sing and dance in front of the mirror. Then she pulls up her T-shirt, right, and then there is this flat stomach and then if I do it, there is this fat one! I mean I would be so happy, if I were Stefanie's size.

Lone: Yes. And then Stefanie still wants to improve something?

Sussie: I think it's because … like Instagram and stuff, people post photos where they are super thin, right? And I think that is what Stefanie is after, where she's just, you know, totally flat [she makes a hand movement in front of her stomach and a sharp sound].

Stefanie: Yes! Thin as a stick!

Sussie: [pointing to herself] And not like this … we call them sex handles! The whole family laughs.

As with Susanne's family, we see here quite different kinds of bodies or weight issues. Does a lump that is hardly noticeable to the outside world qualify as a weight or body concern? Why should Stefanie's little lump get so much attention, even several names? Mette tries to intervene and include here by saying that a small lump can take up a lot of space. The two sisters living at home are very close, and Sussie actually gets it too: she knows that what Stefanie wants is an 'Instagram stomach', totally flat, whereas she herself would be happy if she were Stefanie's size. They both strive for bodily perfections that seem somewhat out of reach. We cannot know what the names and attention given to Stefanie's lump are about: are they about belonging in a family with weight issues? Are they about eliciting special attention and care for being a beautiful changeling? We should be careful not to over-determine the possible explanations in affection (Masquelier et al., this volume). As we saw in Rita's childhood recollection, it can be hard to sort out this sub-social level of the family mud pie (Kuan 2019). However, we can note that both conflicts and care emerge around family body issues.

As the conversation moves on to perceived causes of overweight, the family contemplates structural and historical developments, like fast food chains, family-size bags of crisps and chocolate bars, sedentary work and people driving to the supermarket instead of walking or cycling. Then Mette exclaims: 'I think that if you don't … do something about it, then it goes downhill. Even if you eat normally, reasonably, I mean healthy and a bit unhealthy, then you know – if you do not DO something actively … With the kind of society we have, then you will get too big'. At least, she adds, if you are a family like them, with their kind of genes and appetites, apart from Stefanie, that is, who is a changeling.

This aptly captures the pathic dimension (Waldenfels 2011) of weight gain as something that befalls you, haunts you. Also, we see the affection of place. Sussie notes how she felt thin when she started at her new school, where many people were overweight or obese, and she is also explicit about her own family home as a contagious space, in contrast to the boarding school. In their drawing, several neighbours and friends as well as many family members are obese, which points to issues of social class and inequality in health. Mette's words indicate that 'the kind of society we have' is contagious, and that you have to protect yourself to avoid becoming obese. Just as we have seen affections between people, there are also affections of place (Grøn 2017a; Meinert and Whyte 2017; Solomon 2016; Swinburn et al. 2011).

Configuring Contagious Kinship Connections

I hope in this chapter to have given credit and credibility to Mette's statement that there is so much you have to do in order to avoid becoming obese, if you are part of a family like theirs. I hope to have shown that even though these families subscribe to the individual lifestyle and the energy-expenditure models of obesity, their experiences, drawings and conversations provide a much more complex picture. Families and family members who do overeat do not get obese, and those who do get obese do so in different ways. I hope to have moved convincingly beyond the individual lifestyle explanation that guides most health-related political interventions and is accepted as almost self-explanatory – not only in Denmark but in many parts of the world.

I have drawn on previous work in which I have suggested affection as a phenomenological take on social contagion, which is characterized by indeterminacy and intersubjectivity – features that are central in all four family drawings. However, in this chapter I have highlighted two other dimensions of affection: the deeply affective – yet ambiguous – ties and links that configure affections between people, but also between people and places, genes and family love and hauntings, big hearts and big people. Moreover, that we should talk of obesities in the plural, taking into consideration the specific and particular configurations of affections that make for different kinds of obesity, not only between families but also within them.

Finally, I have sought to demonstrate that phenomenological attention to the lived experience of affection can aid the understanding of how phenomena travel, translate and transform between (often academically) demarcated domains. So that we might begin to grasp how configurations of such diverse affections as senses of self-worth, Danish *hygge*, birth control pills, poverty, childhoods involving sports or not, McDonald's restaurants, gastric bypass surgeries and changelings – and a blue-eyed, curly-haired pop star – intersect and coalesce in biosocial contagion.

Acknowledgements

My heartfelt gratitude goes to the families that I have known for two decades. They have generously shared their experiences and reflections, and I find myself unable to fully convey the richness of their family and obesity stories. I also wish to thank the participants of the EPICENTER group for wonderfully rich and stimulating conversations and collaborations, and the anonymous reviewers who offered very helpful suggestions. Gratitude also to Maria Speyer for never-ceasing inspiration and for allowing me to use her drawing in this chapter. Finally, a special thanks to Lotte Meinert and Jens

Seeberg for organizing, inspiring and leading the EPICENTER project and for editing this book.

Lone Grøn
Professor (WSR)
VIVE – The Danish Center for Social Science Research

Notes

1. Waldenfels' responsive phenomenology (also referred to as phenomenology of the alien) has been used in anthropological studies, mainly to explore radical alienness in phenomena such as spirit possession (Leistle 2014), dreams (Louw 2017) and cen spirits (Meinert and Whyte 2017). I have found his phenomenology equally relevant for the exploration of everyday and ordinary phenomena, such as obesity, in order to move beyond the apparent certainty with which we often think of these things (Grøn 2017a, 2017b, 2020). See also Mattingly (2017, 2018) for an analysis of the alien in the context of the familiar and the intimate.
2. For Maria Speyer's work, see: www.mariaspeyer.com.
3. The genealogical paradigm relies on western ideas of biological and judicial kinship, i.e. kinship through marriage and blood, but also carries specific assumptions and ideas 'concerning sequence, essence, and transmission' (Bamford and Leach 2009: 2).
4. I use pseudonyms for family members in the written text in order to secure anonymity. This means that specific people appearing in the text cannot be identified in the drawings.
5. The use of the word 'it' when pointing out causes of contagion can indicate both uncertainty and doubt in causal pathways (Meinert and Whyte 2017; Williams and Meinert, this volume) and a polyvalent critique, which can be contained within existing family relationships (Meinert 2020).
6 Among their closest friends are Susanne and her husband (from the earlier relatedness drawing). I met both couples at a weight loss programme, when I was carrying out my first period of fieldwork from 2001 to 2003. Since then, a true friendship has evolved between them, they meet often and celebrate birthdays, seasonal parties and so on. Peter and Mette also talk about a 'boom' or an epidemic of gastric bypass surgeries in their network, including Susanne and her two sisters, one of Susanne's friends, two of Peter's colleagues and one of their neighbours.

References

Bamford, Sandra, and James Leach. 2009. *Kinship and Beyond: The Genealogical Model Reconsidered*. New York: Berghahn Books.

Boero, Nathalie. 2007. 'All the News that's Fat to Print: The American "Obesity Epidemic" and the Media', *Qualitative Sociology* 30(1): 41–60.

Carsten, Janet. 2004. *After Kinship*. Cambridge: Cambridge University Press.

Christakis, N.A., and J.H. Fowler. 2007. 'The Spread of Obesity in a Large Social Network over 32 Years', *New England Journal of Medicine* 357: 370–79.

Das, Veena. 1995. 'National Honour and Practical Kinship: Unwanted Women and Children', in Rayna Rapp and Faye Ginsburg (eds), *Conceiving the New World Order: The Global Politics of Reproduction*. Berkeley: University of California Press, pp. 212–33.

Desjarlais, Robert, and Jason C. Throop. 2011. 'Phenomenological Approaches in Anthropology', *Annual Review of Anthropology* 40: 87–102.

Franklin, Sarah, and Susan McKinnon. 2001. 'Introduction', in Sarah Franklin and Susan McKinnon (eds), *Relative Values: Reconfiguring Kinship Studies*. Durham, NC: Duke University Press, pp. 1–25.

Garcia, Angela. 2014. 'Regeneration: Love Drugs, and the Making of Hispano Inheritance', Social Anthropology 22(2): 200–12.

Gard, M., and J. Wright. 2005. *The Obesity Epidemic: Science, Morality and Ideology*. London: Routledge.

Geschiere, Peter. 1997. *The Modernity of Witchcraft: Politics and the Occult in Postcolonial Africa*. Charlottesville: University of Virginia Press.

Greenhalgh, Susan. 2015. *Fat-Talk Nation: The Human Costs of America's War on Fat*. Cornell, NY: Cornell University Press.

Grøn, L. 2017a. 'The Weight of the Family: Communicability as Alien Affection in Danish Family Histories and Experiences of Obesity', *Ethos* 45(2): 182–98.

———. 2017b. 'The Tipping of the Big Stone – And Life Itself: Obesity, Moral Work and Responsive Selves Over Time', *Culture, Medicine, and Psychiatry* 41(2): 267–83.

———. 2020. 'Cutting/Belonging: Sameness and Difference in the Lived Experience of Obesity and Kinship in Denmark', *Ethnos* 85(4): 679–95.

Han, Clara, and Andrew Brandel. 2019. 'Genres of Witnessing: Narrative, Violence, Generations', *Ethnos* 85(4): 629–46.

Hollan, Douglas. 2017. 'Dreamscapes of Intimacy and Isolation: Shadows of Contagion and Immunity', *Ethos* 45(2): 216–31.

Kuan, Teresa. 2019. 'Feelings Run in the Family: Kin Therapeutics and the Configuration of Cause in China', *Ethnos* 85(4): 696–716.

———. Forthcoming. 'Emotion and Affect', in James Laidlaw (ed.), *The Cambridge Handbook for the Anthropology of Ethics and Morality*. Cambridge: Cambridge University Press.

Lambek, Michael. 2011. 'Kinship as Gift and Theft: Acts of Succession in Mayotte and Ancient Israel', *American Ethnologist* 38: 2–16.

Leistle, Bernhard. 2014. 'From the Alien to the Other: Steps Toward a Phenomenological Theory of Spirit Possession', *Anthropology of Consciousness* 25(1): 53–90.

Louw, Maria. 2017. 'Burdening Visions: The Haunting of the Unseen in Bishkek, Kyrgyzstan', *Contemporary Islam* 1–15.

Mattingly, Cheryl. 2017. 'Autism and the Ethics of Care: A Phenomenological Investigation into the Contagion of Nothing', *Ethos* 45(2): 250–70.

———. 2018. 'Ordinary Possibility, Immanent Transcendence and Responsive Ethics: A Philosophical Anthropology of the Small Event', *Hau: Journal of Ethnographic Theory* 8(1–2): 172–84.

Mazzarella, William. 2017. 'Sense out of Sense: Notes on the Affect/Ethics Impasse', *Cultural Anthropology* 32(2): 199–208

McCullough, M.B., and J.A. Hardin. 2013. *Reconstructing Obesity: The Meaning of Measures and the Measure of Meanings*. New York: Berghahn Books.

McKinnon, Susan. 2017. 'Doing and Being: Process, Essence, and Hierarchy in Making Kin', in Simon Coleman, Susan B. Hyatt and Ann Kingsolver (eds), *The Routledge Companion to Contemporary Anthropology*. Abingdon: Routledge, pp. 161–82.

Meinert, Lotte. 2020. 'Haunted Families after the War in Uganda: Doubt as Polyvalent Critique', *Ethnos* 85(4): 595–611.

Meinert, Lotte, and Lone Grøn. 2017. 'Cultural Epidemics and Social Contagion: Phenomenological Approaches', *Ethos* 45(2): 165–81.

———. 2019. 'It Runs in the Family: Exploring Contagious Kinship Connections', *Ethnos* 85(4): 581–94.

Meinert, Lotte, and Susan Reynolds Whyte. 2017. 'These Things Continue: Violence as Contamination in Everyday Life after War in Northern Uganda', *Ethos* 45(2): 271–86.

Moffat, Tina. 2010. 'The Childhood Obesity Epidemic: Health Crisis or Social Construction?', *Medical Anthropology Quarterly* 24(1): 1–21.

Müller-Wille, Staffan, and Hans-Jörg Rheinberger. 2007. *Heredity Produced: At the Crossroads of Biology, Politics, and Culture, 1500–1870*. Cambridge, MA: MIT Press.

Peletz, Michael G. 2001. 'Ambivalence in Kinship since the 1940s', in Sarah Franklin and Susan McKinnon (eds), *Relative Values: Reconfiguring Kinship Studies*. Durham, NC: Duke University Press, pp. 413–44.

Rosa, Hartmut. 2019. *Resonance: A Sociology of Our Relationship to the World*. Cambridge: Polity Press.

Rutherford, Danilyn. 2016. 'Affect Theory and the Empirical', *Annual Review of Anthropology* 45: 285–300.

Sahlins, Marshall. 2013. *What Kinship Is ... And Is Not*. Chicago: University of Chicago Press.

Schneider, David M. 1980. *American Kinship: A Cultural Account*. Chicago: University of Chicago Press.

Seeberg, Jens, and Lotte Meinert. 2015. 'Can Epidemics Be Non-Communicable? Reflections on the Spread of "Non-Communicable" Diseases', *Medicine Anthropology Theory* 2(2): 54–71.
Solomon, H. 2016. *Metabolic Living: Food, Fat, and the Absorption of Illness in India*. Durham, NC: Duke University Press.
Stevenson, Lisa. 2014. *Life Beside Itself: Imagining Care in the Canadian Arctic*. Oakland: University of California Press.
Sørensen, Torben I.A. 2014. 'Challenges in Understanding Development of Obesity', in C. Nobrega and R. Rodriguez-Lopez (eds), *Molecular Mechanisms Underpinning the Development of Obesity*. Cham: Springer, pp. 1–9.
Stasch, R. 2009. *Society of Others: Kinship and Mourning in a West Papuan Place*. Berkeley: University of California Press.
Stewart, K. 2007. *Ordinary Affect*. Durham, NC: Duke University Press.
Swinburn, B.A., et al. 2011. 'The Global Obesity Pandemic: Shaped by Global Drivers and Local Environments', *The Lancet* 378: 804–14.
Viveiros de Castro, E. 2009. 'The Gift and the Given: Three Nano-Essays on Kinship and Magic', in Sandra Bamford and James Leach (eds), *Kinship and Beyond: The Genealogical Model Reconsidered*. Oxford: Berghahn Books, pp. 237–68.
Wagner, R. 1997. 'Analogic Kinship: A Daribi Example', *American Ethnologist* 4(4): 623–42.
Waldenfels, B. 2011. *Phenomenology of the Alien: Basic Concepts*. Evanston, IL: Northwestern University Press.
Whyte, S.R. 1997. *Questioning Misfortune: The Pragmatics of Uncertainty in Eastern Uganda*. Cambridge: Cambridge University Press.
Wright, J., and V. Harwood. 2009. *Bio-politics and the 'Obesity Epidemic': Governing Bodies*. New York: Routledge.

Chapter 5
Health Activists and Trauma Contagion
Cultural Epidemics and Raising Awareness of Trauma in Post-conflict, Post-tsunami Aceh

Jesse Hession Grayman, Mary-Jo DelVecchio Good and Byron J. Good

Introduction

Jens Seeberg and Lotte Meinert (2015), and their colleagues at the EPICENTER, introduced new interpretive prisms to explore and critique standard global health ways of configuring biosocial understandings of non-communicable diseases (NCDs). Susan Whyte's (2012) notion of the spread of social awareness of NCDs is also particularly relevant to a consideration of 'trauma' in environments saturated with high social and political violence and/or massive natural disasters. Lone Grøn and Lotte Meinert, in the introduction to their recent edited journal collection, ask 'how are groups of people affected by similar conditions, even when these are not biologically contagious?' (2017: 165). They note that a variety of NCDs 'have gained global prominence as epidemic problems – diabetes, obesity, trauma, and autism – though [they are] perspectives and concepts from phenomenological and experience near traditions. This includes emic ideas of social contagion and contamination, inter-subjective units of analysis, causal indeterminacy as well as diversity and transformation in social contagion' (ibid.).

We take these comments, which frame and inform this edited volume, as a starting point to revisit our prior studies in post-conflict, post-tsunami Aceh, Indonesia where we and our Acehnese colleagues sought to develop responses that address what we gloss as 'remainders of violence'. This broad term was designed for the International Organization for Migration (IOM) and its global donors to describe the psychosocial needs and mental health disorders we found in our province-wide assessments of high conflict-affected districts. Based on more than a decade of association and collaboration with Acehnese physicians, nurses, public health researchers, university scholars, psychiatrists and psychologists, as well as with the communities served, in this chapter we reflect on the social contagion of trauma and the elevation of trauma from a stigmatizing condition into a shared public concern (M. Good 2010). We focus on the role of Acehnese health professionals, and show ethnographically how they understand trauma's communicability, which in turn motivates their transformation into infectious health activists, manifest in the implementation of innovative mental health interventions. Our narrative strategy in this chapter moves alternately between ethnographic description and social analysis, and highlights our psychosocial needs assessment work and programme intervention with IOM in Aceh that made this inquiry possible (B. Good 2012). We analyse how trauma, conceptualized locally as an epidemic both during and especially after the conflict, influenced the emergence of new and quite robust innovative mental health projects that linked international organizations, government health offices, Indonesian NGOs, clinics and universities to improve care for the mentally ill. We begin with the twin disasters of tsunami and war in Aceh.

Background: Tsunami, Conflict and Mental Health Services in Aceh

On 26 December 2004, a massive earthquake of 9.2 on the Richter scale, reportedly lasting more than ten minutes, struck deep in the sea off the west coast of Aceh province and the provincial capital of Banda Aceh. The earthquake was followed by the great Indian

Ocean Tsunami, with three massive waves rising to thirty metres that swept away 160–180,000 lives almost instantly (and another 60–80,000 in Thailand and Sri Lanka). Tsunami survivors were faced not only with loss of family, homes, belongings and community, but with sites of astonishing devastation and massive debris – crushed houses, wharfs, electrical stations, small boats and large ships, trees, bodies, animals, vehicles – carried by surging ocean waters and deposited two to five kilometres inland, among commercial districts and residential neighbourhoods. Villages, farms and gardens, entire urban areas, and highways and roads were swept away, crumbled, disappeared and destroyed (M. Good, B. Good and Grayman 2010; M. Good and B. Good 2013; Samuels 2019).

A massive international and national humanitarian response followed, with organizations from around the globe and throughout Indonesia arriving to respond to the crisis (B. Good, Grayman and M. Good 2015). The mass entry of international groups into Aceh also brought into global awareness the fierce armed conflict between the Indonesian military of the central government and the Free Aceh Movement (GAM) struggling for political autonomy and most recently for independence, which had persisted for nearly three decades (Aspinall 2009; Drexler 2008; Kell 1995; Reid 2006; Robinson 1998; Siapno 2002). The conflict had profound effects on many rural communities, particularly those up in the hills, away from the tsunami zone, with not only combatants but civilian communities suffering humiliation, torture and killing as well as loss of property and livelihood. The Helsinki Memorandum of Understanding (MOU) of 15 August 2005 brought to conclusion more than a decade of violent conflict, and provided an opening for mental health innovations to move beyond the coastal areas affected by the tsunami to the regions of Aceh that were most affected by the violence (Aguswandi and Large 2008; Aspinall 2005; M. Good and B. Good 2013).

Prior to the tsunami, government-administered mental health care was mostly limited to the provincial psychiatric hospital in Banda Aceh, where the most severely mentally ill were housed, treated and released to homes and families, who were sometimes less than eager to see patients return. The hospital's psychiatrists also provided care through their own robust private practices that catered to many less ill and often more wealthy patients. There were four psychiatrists to treat the entire province of over four million people, and only two were engaged in active medical practice, with few other professionals outside the psychiatric hospital to attend to the mentally ill. The hospital was severely damaged by the tsunami but reopened to hold and care for patients after six months. One psychiatrist left the province. Another was mostly engaged in the hectic immediacy of keeping the hospital running during the post-tsunami era of reconstruction and recovery from the disaster's infrastructural, social and psychological devastation. Of the two practising psychiatrists, one lived three hours away in a neighbouring district and came to direct the hospital four days a week. The other, Dr A, was on the medical faculty of the major state university. He was also the medical director at the psychiatric hospital and reviewed patient medications. He revived his private practice in a small way in the devastated city of Banda Aceh following the tsunami and was recruited by IOM to be the primary consultant on mental health and psychosocial programmes. He was tasked with developing ideas for ways to treat populations traumatized by the tsunami. He offered a decentralized treatment model to IOM – his long-held fantasy about how to build treatment programmes that would reach into the districts and be supported by district hospitals and community health centres (*puskesmas*).

We first met Dr A in June 2005 when we began consulting for IOM on the design of their post-tsunami mental health services. But less than two months later, the peace agreement signalled a major turning point in IOM's (and our) mental health work in Aceh, as IOM secured funding to support the Indonesian government's post-conflict reintegration programme. This included a health component for GAM ex-combatants, amnestied prisoners and conflict-affected communities, and presented IOM with a singular opportunity to assess psychosocial needs in Aceh's previously closed-off conflict areas. The conflict was responsible for the deaths of approximately thirty-five thousand combatants and civilians. While far fewer than the lives lost in the earthquake and tsunami, whole communities experienced aggressive and humiliating violence, displacement and loss of land, destroyed and looted homes and burned public buildings, and grinding, chronic trauma. Conflict survivors thus faced a different type of devastation and traumatic distress than tsunami victims, a kind of trauma that seemed even more difficult to resolve.

By the end of 2005, together with Dr A, IOM's Aceh-based medical team and a team of researchers from Syiah Kuala University, we prepared to launch IOM's post-conflict psychosocial needs assessment (PNA), which led to the design and implementation of programmes to treat populations suffering from conflict-related trauma and other mental disorders. Both the PNA and the interventions were viewed as integral to societal recovery and to build a lasting peace.[1] This is the context in which the ethnographic insights below help us make new sense of our data on trauma as contagion.

Bachtiar: Awakened and Moved by the *Trauma* of Conflict Survivors

Here we introduce another key actor in our work who provided us with insight into how trauma spreads as a productive contagion. Just as our PNA plans were building rapid momentum, we were fortunate to meet Bachtiar in December 2005, immediately after he had been recruited to work at IOM through the United Nations Volunteer (UNV) programme.[2] With formal training in nursing and occupational health, but with practical experience working with torture survivors through a small NGO during the war, Bachtiar's new supervisor at IOM correctly identified him as a good fit with IOM's post-conflict programme. Bachtiar was eager and competent to assist with the PNA, and he quickly became an essential part of our research team.

In an interview with Bachtiar in 2012, we asked what motivated him to work for the NGO RATA (Rehabilitation Action for Torture victims in Aceh) from 1999 to 2003 instead of entering the public health service. He recalled the intake interviews with survivors of violence from the north-eastern districts where the violence was worst at that time: 'When they arrived from their villages in the middle of the night with all of their troubles, we felt moved (*tergugah*) with pity'. *Tergugah* has multivalent meanings that include feeling emotionally moved or touched, but also physically awoken or struck, shaken with realization or awareness. Coming from a rural community not far from Banda Aceh, relatively untouched by the conflict violence, Bachtiar was unaware of how the conflict was affecting ordinary rural communities prior to his work with RATA. These late-night interactions with RATA's patients were career-defining, innocence-shattering moments that persuaded Bachtiar to dedicate his work to trauma recovery and other mental health issues.

Discourses and Phenomenology of *Trauma* in Indonesia and Aceh

Bachtiar's self-conscious awakening and concern with trauma appears to emerge organically from within, born of his concern and support for survivors of torture. But Bachtiar's work with RATA in the early 2000s, with support from international donors, is but one instance of the rapid proliferation of an emergent trauma discourse during that tumultuous period of Indonesia's history. These were the years when trauma programmes were newly featured in the portfolio of post-conflict and humanitarian aid programmes at a global level, especially after the launching of the global war on terror (Breslau 2004). The unique features of an Indonesian understanding of trauma emerged after the fall of President Suharto's authoritarian New Order regime in 1998, embedded in what Dwyer and Santikarma (2007) call 'posttraumatic politics' (cf. B. Good and M. Good 2017). *Trauma* (in Bahasa Indonesia) served as a useful idiom not just for revisiting the once-repressed histories of Suharto's human rights abuses, but also to address the chaotic explosion of political violence across the archipelago – including in Aceh – during the difficult post-authoritarian transition to democracy. The discourse of trauma, with its more clinical connotations, allowed for less overtly political modes of problematizing violence, even as more and more non-clinicians made the diagnosis. But what of the everyday experience of *trauma* in Aceh?

The first thing we learned when talking to people in Aceh about mental health was that *trauma* had been thoroughly absorbed, albeit recently, into everyday understandings of mental illness. One key informant told his interviewer: 'Before the conflict, no one around here knew the word *trauma*'. But what did this mean in the context of post-conflict Aceh? An extremely common initial presentation of distress, reflected in our interviews, in clinical interactions and in the medical records, would begin with a simple statement, *jantung berdebar debar*, my heart pounds.[3] Those diagnosed as suffering from a psychiatric disorder would often go on: *Saya sering takut*, I am often afraid. *Teringat*, I have memories that come unbidden to me. *Tidak bisa tidur dengan enak*, I can't sleep well at night; *terbangun*, I wake up feeling frightened, and cannot sleep again. *Gelisah*, I often feel restless, anxious, worried. My body feels weak, *lemah*; I lack spirit or energy, *semangat*, so that I am unable to go off to work in the rice paddies or the gardens. These are some of the symptoms that characterize a local phenomenology of trauma-related illnesses in Aceh (B. Good and M. Good 2017; B. Good, M. Good and Grayman 2016; M. Good 2010).

We found it useful to contrast local understandings of *trauma* with another word imported from English: *stres* (from stress). The meanings of *stres* and *trauma* overlap, both denoting deep psychological distress brought on by external events such as war, a death in the family or a natural disaster, but we learned through interviews and everyday conversation that in Aceh *trauma* is considered a temporary condition from which one can recover. In contrast, the word *stres* – unlike in English, where stress might suggest something as light as the effects of a bad day at the office – denotes a more serious, long-term condition that may require psychiatric care at a hospital. One might be suffering from *trauma* but still be present and functional in the community, whereas when someone has *stres*, he or she is noticeably debilitated from performing everyday social roles. The word *trauma* tends to appear more often in everyday conversation (e.g. 'Everyone in this village still has *trauma* from the conflict') (Grayman, M. Good and B. Good 2009). Catherine Smith's recent ethnography on the localization of trauma in Aceh (2018) broadly validates these findings, and she goes further to show how everyday deployment of the word *trauma* can have a communal, protective effect on vulnerable individuals or groups in order to minimize the stigma associated with more serious forms of mental illness such as *stres*, or *pungo*, the Acehnese word for crazy.

Local understandings of *trauma* in Aceh do not precisely match either the clinical psychiatric definition for PTSD or global humanitarian aid organizations' understanding of trauma. Despite these differences in how diverse stakeholders define and understand trauma/ *trauma*, Smith (2018) follows Fassin and Rechtman (2009) in arguing that the trauma discourse productively problematizes violence, albeit in different modes. During the first few years of the peace process in Aceh, there was sufficient overlap in the apprehension of trauma among a diverse array of stakeholders – survivors, activists, humanitarians, clinicians, government officials, academics, journalists and politicians – to productively leverage the concept for Aceh's recovery from war. IOM's PNA and subsequent intervention illustrate how these stakeholders turned a study of trauma and other psychological burdens into a critique of the 'remainders of violence' in post-conflict Aceh.

The IOM Psychosocial Needs Assessment

In November 2005, IOM invited us to help design and oversee the conduct of a 'psychosocial needs assessment' (PNA) in high-conflict subdistricts of three districts of Aceh that had been most affected by the violence (Bireuen, Aceh Utara and Pidie). The needs assessment was aimed at guiding the development of IOM psychosocial and mental health programmes. The goal was to evaluate levels of traumatic events associated with the conflict, levels of psychological and psychiatric symptoms, levels of disability associated with mental health conditions, and desire for particular kinds of services. Working with teams from IOM and Aceh's Syiah Kuala University, surveys were conducted to provide data from a representative sample of adults (n=596) in villages in high-conflict subdistricts in the three districts on Aceh's north coast in February 2006. When the initial study (described as PNA1, see B. Good et al. 2006) was found to be highly significant in seeking funding and carrying out mental health programmes, IOM secured eager donor support to expand the needs assessment to a similar sample of adults (n=1,376) in eleven more districts around Aceh in July 2006 (described as PNA2, see M. Good et al. 2007).

Using a 43-item Harvard Trauma Events scale, adapted specifically to represent typical forms of trauma experienced in rural communities across Aceh, the surveys found shockingly high levels of conflict-related traumatic experiences, particularly in Aceh's north, east and southwest regions. These included experiences of combat, firefights, bombing, beatings, humiliation, torture, destruction of houses, lands and animals, loss of spouses and children, and loss of freedom to work, to farm their lands or tend to their businesses or send children to school, or to cross the street, to travel to the cities, to Banda Aceh or Medan on a bus or in a private car. In high-conflict areas, 78–80 per cent of adults experienced combat, 48–66 per cent of men reported being beaten, and 24–25 per cent of men reported being tortured. Women experienced lower rates of physical violence than men, but rates for women were also extraordinarily high. For example, in the PNA1 subdistricts, 20 per cent of women reported being beaten (compared with 56 per cent of men) and 11 per cent reported being tortured (compared with 25 per cent of men). There were also extremely high rates of head trauma, associated with interrogation and violence against community members. In the PNA1 samples, 41 per cent of men and 12 per cent of women reported being beaten to the head or suffocated, which in some cases led to permanent brain damage. In one district, 68 per cent of young men aged seventeen to twenty-nine reported such head trauma.

The surveys also documented extraordinarily high rates of psychological symptoms, comparable to those in war zones such as Bosnia. Using standard, international symptom checklists, adapted for use in Aceh, the surveys found levels of anxiety, depression and PTSD symptoms that were extraordinarily high. For example, in the PNA1 study, using international levels for rating 'high' levels of symptoms, 64 per cent of men and 67 per cent of women suffered high levels of depressive symptoms, 64 per cent of men and 75 per cent of women high anxiety symptoms, and 33 per cent of men and 35 per cent of women high levels of symptoms of PTSD. These symptoms were highly and directly related to numbers of traumatic events individuals had suffered. The PNA2 surveys, conducted five months later when more of the special forces had left Aceh, found significantly lower overall rates of symptoms, suggesting that symptom levels did not necessarily represent mental illness. However, levels continued to show high associations with levels of traumatic events.[4] Thus, the study showed that mental health symptoms (formal diagnoses were not made in the survey) were indeed 'epidemic' in the communities that experienced high levels of violence, and these symptoms were much higher among those who suffered higher levels of traumatic violence.

Trauma Contagion

PNA respondents often experienced unexpected relief upon sharing their traumatic experiences with their interviewers. 'No one ever asked us about what happened here' was a frequent refrain.

Karlina Supelli, a philosophy lecturer at a Jesuit college in Jakarta who came to prominence for her activism on behalf of Chinese-Indonesian sexual assault survivors of the 1998 riots, describes such sharing as *mengalihan sengsara*, to redirect one's suffering outside the self by putting experience into words and out of one's head (M. Good, B. Good and Grayman 2010). The research staff evocatively described the process of listening. They used the phrase *melampiaskan penderitaan* to describe respondents' conflict stories, which means to 'release one's suffering'. The verb *melampiaskan* has a physical, rushing, flowing, even an explosive or sexual connotation, frequently associated with anger and lust, and almost always takes an object, which is to say that the research staff were the receptacles of their respondents' redirected suffering. The researchers found this transfer of suffering difficult and exhausting, and team leaders found it helpful to set aside some recreation time for their researcher-interviewers to process the burden.

Not unlike Bachtiar when he began working with RATA, many of the researchers – all of whom were Acehnese, but mostly from urban areas – were visiting conflict-affected villages in Aceh for the first time. For many, learning about the experiences of ordinary civilians who lived through multiple traumatic events was a shocking revelation. During the PNA1, when Indonesian security forces had left their occupation posts in every village only weeks before our arrival, and the success of the nascent peace was hardly guaranteed, the staff were even fearful of the 'poisonous knowledge' they had acquired from trauma survivors (Das 2000). Several sought reassurances that their names would not appear in our published reports as participants in the research.

After the PNA fieldwork, we and our research teams had opportunities to process and reflect upon this transfer of 'poisonous knowledge'. While doing data entry and transcribing interviews, Bachtiar complained daily of headaches, obviously burdened by the stories he was tasked with preserving in our data archive. Our more experienced team leaders pronounced in one forum after another that their work on the PNA was by far the hardest research they had ever undertaken. We, the chapter authors, variously reported having nightmares and sleepless nights throughout 2006 and 2007. We broadly describe all of this with the label 'secondary trauma'; this is hardly a new phenomenon, we are not surprised by it, nor do we romanticize it. But we highlight it here as the trauma contagion, the phenomenological experience of learning to live with poisonous or traumatic knowledge, albeit secondary and diluted, that adds purchase to the emergent trauma discourse across Indonesia, as it travels from rural to urban, and transfers from Aceh's ordinary survivors of violence to Aceh's professional elites. In the remainder of this chapter, we describe the successful intervention that these difficult research findings supported, and we argue that the very success of this programme and others like it turned upon the determination and motivation of 'trauma activists' like Bachtiar.

The IOM Model of Providing Mental Health Outreach Services

The PNA data confirmed that villagers had a strong desire for mental health services, as well as for other forms of support, but that powerful memories of the surveillance of the health care system by the military were preventing them from seeking treatment. Acehnese are resilient, and many recovered over time without medical forms of mental health care. However, many continued to show signs of classic PTSD, of reliving terrible events they had witnessed or experienced, with associated nightmares, panic attacks and anxiety, as well as elevated rates of depression, sleep disorders and disabling anxiety.

We worked closely with IOM and district health offices to develop a model that could provide services for adults in the community with common or more severe mental health problems to particularly high-conflict and relatively isolated villages on an emergency basis, while building capacity within the primary health care system. A small group of dedicated Acehnese general practitioners and nurses – who were selected because they were among the most committed clinicians working in other IOM programmes – were recruited and given short, specialized training and close supervision by an Acehnese psychiatrist. They formed mobile mental health outreach teams, who along with community mental health nurses (CMHNs)[5] from the nearest *puskesmas*, went into villages, provided general medical care, sought out persons with mental health problems, and provided treatment – including diagnosis and medication, counselling and family visits, the formation of village-level support groups, and in a subset of villages, 'livelihood' support. Throughout all stages, the Acehnese doctors and nurses, along with support staff, played strategic roles such as the selection of villages to include for outreach, advocacy with local authorities, and promoting the programme through videos and lectures to local audiences.

The intervention with IOM included a rigorous evaluation. We report a detailed review of this evaluation in B. Good, M. Good and Grayman (2016), but provide a few highlights here. First, the intervention demonstrated that competent mental health care could be provided by GPs and nurses making monthly visits to villages, and, consistent with what we learned during the assessment, that such services would be strongly supported by local communities. Second, the research demonstrated that overall, rates of recovery were remarkably high, for both men and women. Of those who completed the outcome study, 83 per cent reported some to great improvement in their symptoms. The percent of persons with high levels of anxiety symptoms dropped from 90 per cent before treatment to 54 per cent after treatment; those with high levels of PTSD symptoms were reduced from 26 per cent to 8 per cent; and those with high levels of depressive symptoms dropped from 73 per cent to 38 per cent. Third, the project demonstrated that common mental health disorders are terribly disabling, and that treatment is extremely powerful in returning individuals to regular work and social functioning. When individuals entered treatment, they reported that before they became ill, they were able to work on average twenty-eight hours per week (even though limited by the conflict); when they fell ill, this was reduced to ten hours per week. At the end of treatment, individuals reported that they could now work an average forty-one hours per week! Meanwhile, the patients who participated in the experimental 'livelihood' component (approximately 20 per cent, n=200) showed highly significant improvements in the way they rated their levels of symptoms, as well as their ability to work.

Trauma Activists

Post-disaster mental health interventions such as the IOM programme described here and the CMHN programme not only resulted in the delivery of urgently needed care in a humanitarian context, but also trained new cadres of Acehnese and Indonesian activists empowered to carry this work forward throughout Indonesia. The mundane building of mental health teams and treatment programmes and assessing outcomes and debating policies with government stakeholders – excited, supportive, but also hard and competitive – produced, in fact, a kind of cultural and social movement. We discerned an innovation in perception of the importance of mental health work, and a desire, positive and inspirational at times, to help those suffering not only from 'trauma' – the collective experiences of so many Acehnese – but also from severe mental disorders, from psychoses to severe depression or extreme anxiety and panic and PTSD disorders, often in isolated settings and with little care. The young physicians, nurses, psychologists and researchers participated in the mundane activities of health systems development and care as willing and even eager participants in a social and cultural shift, a sequela arising from post-conflict interventions, which they designed and implemented to care for their fellow Acehnese who suffered various degrees of trauma during the conflict.

In a setting where the vast majority of Acehnese had lived through traumatic experiences – due to tsunami, conflict or both – or knew close friends or family who had, professionals and patients empathized with each other. It may well have been this empathy that led to an expansion of psychiatrists in Aceh. By 2013, the number of psychiatrists had risen to 15–17 in the province, with over ten in Banda Aceh and several located in the major district community hospitals. Many of these psychiatrists are women; most are Acehnese. Psychologists as well, also mostly women, began to be integrated into the mental health treatment programmes slowly developing in the *puskesmas*.

We argue that empathy for and identification with those who suffered trauma allowed health professionals to reduce their fear and stigma towards persons living with severe mental illnesses. Indeed, many of those who lived with the remainders of violence or the devastation from the tsunami were in serious need of care and treatment. A new generation of young health professionals applied their newly acquired knowledge and skills to work towards new models of better care for the severely mentally ill. Indeed, the first post-conflict democratic election for governor brought to power Irwandi Yusuf, a former GAM leader who in 2007 declared – around the same time that our research findings with IOM received significant attention in the local press – that the severely mentally ill should be provided with proper mental health care and be freed from restraints. An alternative political reality was wed to mental health innovations and practice (B. Good, M. Good and Grayman 2019; Puteh, Marthoenis and Minas 2011; Smith 2018).

Recent scholarship on brokerage in Indonesia's health sector highlights the important and effective role brokers play in situating health services (such as Indonesia's new national health insurance scheme) within familiar, personal networks to make them more accessible (Berenschot, Hanani and Sambodho 2018). Indeed, one of the priority goals of IOM's intervention in collaboration with local district health offices was to reintroduce conflict survivors to government health services after generations of conflict had totally alienated civilians from availing themselves of any government services. Health brokers such as Bachtiar and the others working on the IOM team took a leading role in mediating the repair of these connections, though in our work they preferred to call themselves 'activists'. In the aid sector, the best brokers are highly sought by donor agencies and NGOs, for they are uniquely situated to understand, support and advocate for policies and programmes that reflect donor agendas. In the more specific setting of post-conflict recovery programmes in Aceh, health brokers well-versed in an Indonesian politics of connection ultimately performed important acts of reintegration. At first, they authoritatively delivered programmes with generous international funding in a way that met a humanitarian demand, in this case the post-conflict trauma identified in such stark figures in IOM's PNA. The IOM doctors, nurses and psychiatrists who participated in this work passionately and aggressively pressed IOM leadership to respond to the high levels of violence and associated psychiatric distress they witnessed. But just as important, in their efforts to reintroduce civilian communities to government health services, these health activists also had to coordinate with and secure support from local and national government agencies, in this case the local district health offices and *puskesmas* clinics, with whom they forged particularly close working relationships. In former conflict areas, this included coordination with Indonesian security forces, which IOM's research teams, doctors and nurses all successfully navigated. The programmes that non-profit sector activists delivered ultimately bore the imprimatur of not just their international donors, but also the Indonesian central government (Grayman 2013). Such recognition does not quite imply government admission of culpability for political violence of the past, but does perhaps suggest that an attenuated trauma contagion, spread through the dedicated work of health activists, persuaded government health actors to acknowledge and treat people and communities with care instead of denial. This was often discussed in terms of the need for 'trauma healing'.

Conclusion

Our perspective is influenced by our Acehnese medical and research colleagues who were involved in providing succour and healing to communities and individuals living with conflict-induced trauma, which in certain regions produced a vicious collective cultural trauma (Alexander et al. 2004; Eyerman 2001; Kerr Chiovenda 2016). Our colleagues in Aceh willingly took on the contagious burden of this collective trauma, then mobilized their social and political capital, and expertise, to address it. They elevated the suffering of individuals and communities that still live with the remainders of violence in Aceh into a shared, public concern by way of trauma and trauma-related diagnoses and discourses. They are 'trauma brokers' not just in the sense of older anthropological understandings of brokerage, as cultural translators who vernacularize global and national institutions, programmes and services for local populations; they are also agentive, strategic actors who make meaning and foster connections through their practice (Lewis and Mosse 2006).

Concern for the mental health of conflict and tsunami survivors in Aceh has translated into greater awareness of mental health issues – particularly psychosis – than ever seen before, evidenced by the increased reporting in newspapers, frequent pronouncements of concern from local and provincial politicians, the growth of public mental health care and the continuation of the Community Mental Health Nursing programme. The 'Aceh Model' has influenced the development of programmes nationally (B. Good, M. Good and Grayman 2019). From 2010 to 2014, psychiatrists and psychologists from the Faculty of Medicine at Syiah Kuala University collaborated with district health programmes on action-oriented research and intervention programmes to tighten the links between the major provincial university and district governments in introducing and evaluating new practices in public mental health.[6] Today these professionals work on issues more mundane but no less challenging than post-conflict trauma interventions, attempting to provide quality care to the severely and seriously mentally ill by building new systems of professional education and clinical practice (B. Good, M. Good and Grayman 2019). Our ethnography in this chapter shows how the 'trauma contagion' played an important role in raising awareness, concern and ultimately support for these broader mental health service delivery concerns in Aceh, and arguably across Indonesia. And it suggests that by reframing mental health problems in moral and political terms, the word 'trauma' led to recognition of the 'epidemic' quality of post-conflict suffering and helped reduce stigma associated with mental illnesses and their treatment in the Acehnese context.

While these significant developments in mental health care in Aceh leave us cautiously optimistic, our discussions with mental health professionals indicate that the promise of these innovations has not been realized to the extent it was hoped at the time of the most active developments during the post-tsunami and post-conflict periods. *Puskesmas* staff are burdened by a growing number of programmes, particularly since the launch of Indonesia's national health insurance scheme. Formal budgets for mental health services at the national, provincial, district and *puskesmas* levels are often lacking. Mental health remains a limited priority throughout most of the country. This work thus remains incomplete.

Jesse Hession Grayman
Senior Lecturer, Development Studies
School of Social Sciences, Faculty of Arts, University of Auckland, Aotearoa New Zealand.

Mary-Jo DelVecchio Good
Professor Emeritus, Department of Global Health and Social Medicine
Harvard Medical School, Harvard University, USA.

Jesse Hession Grayman, Mary-Jo DelVecchio Good and Byron J. Good

Byron J. Good
Professor of Medical Anthropology
Department of Global Health and Social Medicine, Harvard Medical School, and Department of Anthropology, Harvard University

Notes

1. The 'we' throughout this chapter refers to the three authors, but in differing configurations. Mary-Jo and Byron Good were first invited to consult with IOM about developing mental health responses to the tsunami. Jesse Hession Grayman, at the time a PhD student, joined IOM as an intern, then remained to work as a member of the IOM staff. When IOM contracted with the Goods and Harvard to conduct the psychosocial needs assessment, Grayman joined the project as coordinator for IOM. The three of us continued to collaborate throughout the programme, though the Goods were more directly involved in the intervention project that followed than Grayman.
2. Names of our Acehnese colleagues, their patients and other interlocutors in Aceh are pseudonyms unless directly identified.
3. This analysis reports symptoms in Bahasa Indonesia, or Indonesian language. Local villages in our region spoke primarily Acehnese. The Indonesian terms here are translations of Acehnese and the terms used when Acehnese spoke Indonesian.
4. For a more detailed methodological discussion of how the Harvard Trauma Questionnaire and symptom checklists were used to estimate levels of depression, anxiety and PTSD, see the PNA1 and PNA2 reports (B. Good et al. 2006; M. Good et al. 2007).
5. The Community Mental Health Nursing programme is another important and innovative programme introduced in Aceh after the tsunami to support mental health services in tsunami-affected communities. IOM's post-conflict mental health programme supported the training of additional CMHNs in conflict-affected areas of two districts. See B. Good, M. Good and Grayman (2016) for more about the innovations and limitations of the CMHN model, as well as a more detailed review of the impact evaluation of IOM's outreach programme.
6. This work was supported by a USAID grant, 'Inter-University Partnerships for Strengthening Health Systems in Indonesia: Building New Capacity for Mental Health Care', linking Harvard Medical School, Gadjah Mada University and Syiah Kuala University (Cooperative Agreement No. AID-497-A-11-00015).

References

Aguswandi and J. Large (eds). 2008. *Accord, Reconfiguring Politics: The Indonesia-Aceh Peace Process*. London: Conciliation Resources.

Alexander, J.C., et al. 2004. *Cultural Trauma and Collective Identity*. Berkeley: University of California Press.

Aspinall, Edward. 2005. *The Helsinki Agreement: A More Promising Basis for Peace in Aceh?* Policy Studies No. 20. Washington, DC: East-West Center Washington.

——— 2009. *Islam and Nation: Separatist Rebellion in Aceh, Indonesia*. Stanford, CA: Stanford University Press.

Barter, Shane. 2004. *Neither Wolf, Nor Lamb: Embracing Civil Society in the Aceh Conflict*. Bangkok: Forum Asia.

Berenschot, Ward, Retna Hanani and Prio Sambodho. 2018. 'Brokers and Citizenship: Access to Health Care in Indonesia', *Citizenship Studies* 22(2): 129–44.

Breslau, J. 2004. 'Introduction. Cultures of Trauma: Anthropological Views of Posttraumatic Stress Disorder in International Health', *Culture, Medicine, and Psychiatry* 28(2): 113–26.

Das, Veena. 2000. 'The Act of Witnessing: Violence, Poisonous Knowledge, and Subjectivity', in Veena Das, Arthur Kleinman, Mamphela Ramphele and Pamela Reynolds (eds), *Violence and Subjectivity*. Berkeley: University of California Press, pp. 205–25.

Drexler, Elizabeth F. 2008. *Aceh, Indonesia: Securing the Insecure State*. Philadelphia: University of Pennsylvania Press.

Dwyer, Leslie, and Degung Santikarma. 2007. 'Posttraumatic Politics: Violence, Memory, and Biomedical Discourse in Bali', in L. Kirmayer, R. Lemelson and M. Barad (eds), *Understanding Trauma*. New York: Cambridge University Press, pp. 403–32.

Eyerman, R. 2001. *Cultural Trauma: Slavery and the Formation of African American Identity*. Cambridge: Cambridge University Press.

Fassin, D., and R. Rechtman. 2009. *The Empire of Trauma: An Inquiry into the Condition of Victimhood*, trans. R. Gomme. Princeton, NJ: Princeton University Press.

Good, Byron. J. 2012. 'Theorizing the "Subject" of Medical and Psychiatric Anthropology', *Journal of the Royal Anthropological Institute* 18(3): 515–35.

Good, Byron J., and Mary-Jo DelVecchio Good. 2017. 'Toward a Cultural Psychology of Trauma and Trauma-Related Disorders', in Julia A. Cassaniti and Usha Menon (eds), *Universalism without Universalism*. Chicago: University of Chicago Press, pp. 260–79.

Good, Byron J., Mary-Jo DelVecchio Good and Jesse Hession Grayman. 2016. 'Is PTSD a "Good Enough" Concept for Post-Conflict Mental Health Work? Reflections on Work in Aceh, Indonesia', in Devon E. Hinton and Byron J. Good (eds), *Culture and PTSD: Trauma in Global and Historical Perspective*. Philadelphia: University of Pennsylvania Press, pp. 387–417.

——— 2019. 'Mereka-ulang Perawatan Kesehatan Jiwa Pasca-Tsunami dan Pasca Konflik Aceh' [Reimagining Mental Health Care in Post-Tsunami, Post-Conflict Aceh], in Hans Pols et al. (eds), *Jiwa Sehat, Negara Kuat: Masa Depan Layanan Kesehatan Jiwa di Indonesia*, vol 1. Jakarta: Penerbit Buku KOMPAS, pp. 7–40.

Good, Byron J., Jesse Hession Grayman and Mary-Jo DelVecchio Good. 2015. 'Humanitarianism and "Mobile Sovereignty" in Strong State Settings: Reflections on Medical Humanitarianism in Aceh, Indonesia', in Sharon Abramowitz and Catherine Panter-Brick (eds), *Medical Humanitarianism: Ethnographies of Practice*. Philadelphia: University of Pennsylvania Press, pp. 155–75.

Good, Byron J., et al. 2006. *Psychosocial Needs Assessment of Communities Affected by the Conflict in the Districts of Pidie, Bireuen and Aceh Utara*. Jakarta: International Organization for Migration.

Good, Mary-Jo DelVecchio. 2010. 'Trauma in Postconflict Aceh and Psychopharmaceuticals as a Medium of Exchange', in Janis H. Jenkins (ed.), *The Pharmaceutical Self: The Global Shaping of Experience in an Age of Psychopharmacology*. Santa Fe: SAR Press, pp. 41–66.

Good, Mary-Jo DelVecchio, and Byron J. Good. 2013. 'Perspectives on the Politics of Peace in Aceh, Indonesia', in Felicity Aulino et al. (eds), *Radical Egalitarianism*. New York: Fordham University Press, pp. 191–208.

Good, Mary-Jo DelVecchio, Byron J. Good and Jesse Grayman. 2010. 'Complex Engagements: Responding to Violence in Postconflict Aceh', in Didier Fassin and Mariella Pandolfi (eds), *Contemporary States of Emergency: The Politics of Military and Humanitarian Interventions*. New York: Zone Books, pp. 241–66.

Good, Mary-Jo DelVecchio, et al. 2007. *A Psychosocial Needs Assessment of Communities in 14 Conflict-Affected Districts in Aceh*. Jakarta: International Organization for Migration.

Grayman, Jesse Hession. 2013. 'Humanitarian Encounters in Post-Conflict Aceh, Indonesia', Ph.D. dissertation. Harvard University.

Grayman, Jesse Hession, Mary-Jo DelVecchio Good and Byron J. Good. 2009. 'Conflict Nightmares and Trauma in Aceh', *Culture, Medicine, and Psychiatry* 33(2): 290–312.

Grøn, Lone, and Lotte Meinert. 2017. 'Social Contagion and Cultural Epidemics: Phenomenological and "Experience-Near" Explorations', *Ethos* 45(2): 165–81.

Kell, Tim. 1995. *The Roots of Acehnese Rebellion, 1989–1992*. Ithaca, NY: Cornell Modern Indonesia Project, Southeast Asia Program, Cornell University.

Kerr Chiovenda, Melissa S. 2016. 'Cultural Trauma, History Making, and the Politics of Ethnic Identity among Afghan Hazaras', Ph.D. dissertation. University of Connecticut, https://opencommons.uconn.edu/dissertations/1324.

Lewis, David, and David Mosse. 2006. 'Theoretical Approaches to Brokerage and Translation in Development', in David Lewis and David Mosse (eds),

Development Brokers and Translators: Ethnography of Aid and Agencies. Bloomfield: Kumarian Press, pp. 1–26.

Puteh, Ibrahim, M. Marthoenis and Harry Minas. 2011. 'Aceh Free Pasung: Releasing the Mentally Ill from Physical Restraint', *International Journal of Mental Health Systems* 5: 1–5.

Reid, Anthony (ed.). 2006. *Verandah of Violence: The Background to the Aceh Problem*. Singapore: Singapore University Press.

Robinson, Geoffrey. 1998. 'Rawan is as Rawan Does: The Origins of Disorder in New Order Aceh', *Indonesia* 66: 127–57.

Samuels, Annemarie. 2019. *After the Tsunami: Disaster Narratives and the Remaking of Everyday Life in Aceh*. Honolulu: University of Hawai i Press.

Seeberg, Jens, and Lotte Meinert. 2015. 'Can Epidemics be Noncommunicable? Reflections on the Spread of "Noncommunicable" Diseases', *Medicine Anthropology Theory* 2(2): 54–71.

Siapno, Jacqueline Aquino. 2002. *Gender, Islam, Nationalism and the State in Aceh: The Paradox of Power, Co-optation and Resistance*. London: Routledge.

Smith, Catherine. 2018. *Resilience and the Localisation of Trauma in Aceh, Indonesia*. Singapore: National University of Singapore Press.

Whyte, Susan Reynolds. 2012. 'Chronicity and Control: Framing Noncommunicable Diseases in Africa', *Anthropology and Medicine* 19(1): 63–74.

Chapter 6
Touched by Violence
Configuring Affliction after War in Northern Uganda
Lars Williams and Lotte Meinert

Alfred's Brother

In a clay hut in northern Uganda two brothers are quarrelling. It is a Thursday evening in 1997. Darkness is falling over the camp for internally displaced persons (IDPs), making the grass-thatched roofs of the tightly packed huts stand out clearly against the evening sky. The two brothers are angry. They are both young, muscular men, with bodies shaped by the hard physical work in the fields they have shared since childhood. The older brother James[1] is fed up with the government and the way it has been treating the Acholi people. He is ready to rebel. He wants to join the ranks of the Lord's Resistance Army and fight in the bush. And he wants his younger brother Alfred to join him, so they can fight the injustice together. But Alfred does not want to go. He does not think that more violence is the answer to the situation.

The older brother James joins the rebel army that night. Two days n, or covers his body. As if something from the outside has made its way inside him. He starts to become more aggressive, shouting at people walking by and threatening them. He becomes aggressive towards family members and friends. He occasionally stops eating and drinking, and begins to wander. He wanders around the village, to the trading centre, and often he does not recognize his family members and friends when they see him there. His mother Beatrice tells us that one morning Alfred burst into his parents' house. Here he stood and looked at them for a while like a stranger and suddenly started to laugh out loud. His younger sister, who was only around six years old at the time, remembers that Alfred would yell and scream at night so her other brothers would have to come and hold him down until he calmed down. Alfred starts to see visions of armed men with rifles and machetes following him. He dreams about his dead brother in the bush, his mother explains to us. He had become what in Acholi language is called *lapoya*, a mad person, and sometimes his madness is so fierce that his brothers have to tie him down in their hut.

This chapter is based on anthropological fieldwork in northern Uganda in 2014–16, with follow-up interviews in 2019. Lotte Meinert met Alfred's mother Beatrice in 2014 during a study of trauma and spirits. This study included nineteen families, two health clinics, and interviews with traditional healers, NGOs and clergy. Alfred's mother described the family's and her son's affliction from the perspective of a parent. Later Meinert met Alfred's sister, and finally interviewed Alfred himself in 2015 and again in 2019. Lars Williams lived with Alfred's family at the beginning of 2016 as part of his PhD fieldwork about how mental illness is managed in northern Uganda, with a focus on the Pentecostal-Charismatic churches. It was with a point of departure in Alfred's family that Williams started his study of the Acholi language and of religious practices in relation to mental illness. Williams participated in everyday life with Alfred and his family and kept in contact over two years. Alfred and his family have been a central case in the ethnographic studies we have both carried out in northern Uganda.

Alfred's case is presented in this chapter as it unfolds over a number of years, based on the extended case method (Gluckman 1961; Van Velsen 2017), with a view to focusing on nuances, different positions and changes over time.[2]

The LRA War and Its Aftermath

Two generations of Acholi people in northern Uganda have lived through brutal wars. Many have been subjected to violence and massacres perpetrated not only by the rebel group the Lord's Resistance

Army, but also by Ugandan government soldiers (UPDF) between 1986 and 2006. In the 1990s, the government soldiers placed the majority of the population in IDP camps. Here many lived under conditions that have been described as 'social torture' (Dolan 2008). Over roughly twenty years, experiences of violence, abuse and mistrust structured relations between neighbours (Meinert 2015). The rates of PTSD and depression in northern Uganda are among the highest in the world (Amone-P'Olak, Dokkedahl and Elklit 2017). Suicide rates are high, particularly among young men (Oboke and Whyte 2019; Whyte and Oboke, this volume). Although statistics of mental illness from the region should probably be taken with a grain of salt, there is no doubt that poor mental health is a major problem in northern Uganda.

Since the cessation of hostilities agreement in 2007, the region has been relatively stable in military terms, and people are recovering their everyday lives and relationships. However, new problems have arisen in the aftermath of the conflict and violence. Alcoholism, domestic violence, land conflicts, mental illness and physical disabilities are all widespread problems touching the lives of many. The years of violence have created a legacy which keeps transforming into new problems in the lives of the people in the Acholi region (Meinert and Whyte 2020). Many new actors and organizations have found a space in the post-conflict landscape, bringing promises of hope and healing. The old Catholic and Anglican churches, which had a religious monopoly for many years, now feel challenged by a myriad of Pentecostal-Charismatic churches which have become popular in the region as they have elsewhere in the world (Robbins 2004). Traditional healers (*ajwaki*), hospitals with doctors and biomedicine, along with the many foreign humanitarian and development organizations, also offer alternatives to the state and church. NGOs offering various kinds of psychosocial treatment and trauma therapy have become more common. The many options are negotiated, tried out, combined in a myriad of ways, and often abandoned (Meinert and Whyte 2020).

When the effects of years of violence are placed within particular therapeutic frameworks, they indicate a direction for action. When they are conceptualized as post-traumatic stress disorder (PTSD), spirit possession or something else, experiences are shaped through language and practice – pointing towards specific paths of treatment and recovery. One could, as Fassin and Rechtman suggest, focus on the spread of labels and diagnoses from the Global North to the rest of the world, as they do in their book *Empire of Trauma* (2009), and examine how diagnoses shape experience and practice. It is no coincidence that these labels and discourses spread in particular locations. Diagnoses often come with and give access to resources, where these are scarce, *and* violence creates fragility and susceptibility enabling these discourses, diagnoses and labels to resonate. Even so, people are not always interested in labels even though they have been afflicted by violence. Some people, like Alfred, whose family had experienced violence, were not interested in labels – least of all in a PTSD label. For this reason, we focus beyond the spread of diagnoses and look at the spread of violence and treatment. Violence and its legacies continue to transform and contaminate northern Uganda, causing afflictions and ruptures in everyday lives (Meinert and Whyte 2017). The concept of affliction (Das 2015) is adopted to point to the sense of endurance and pragmatism with which people approach their problems. The actors and institutions mentioned above create spaces in which people try to deal with the legacies of violence: in family life, in trauma therapy, through prayer in church and with biomedicine at the hospital. These arenas of interpretation and healing are not separate and distinct systems, but largely overlapping arenas in which people try out possibilities in a pragmatic and subjunctive mood (Whyte 1997). With the concepts of contagion, contamination and configuring, and the notion of touch, we explore how experiences of violence interplay with institutions in shaping the afflictions that families live with and attempt to manage. Instead of examining separate healing systems – like traditional healing, Christian churches or psychotherapeutic organizations – we examine how these systems continuously intertwine and influence each other, creating new ways of understanding affliction and new paths for action. For this reason, we begin with Alfred's experience of violence: the encounter with the pile of dead bodies through which he had to dig to find his brother James. This violence is the primary phenomenon creating the affliction that haunts Alfred and the family. We follow Alfred and his family into the various institutions which address the consequences of violence and offer treatment and therapy from their various perspectives.

Lars Williams and Lotte Meinert

With Touch: Social Contagion, Contamination and Configuring as Analytical Concepts

A critical phenomenological and practice-oriented approach guides our exploration of the systemic configurations in which problems with spirits and trauma emerge. We take up medical historian Rosenberg's concepts of contamination, contagion and configuration (1992), using them not to describe historical periods, as he does, but as analytical perspectives (Seeberg and Meinert 2015) to describe and understand these systemic processes.

Here *social contagion* refers to processes in which something is transmitted from one actor to another; someone is touched physically, socially, spiritually or otherwise, and is affected by this touching.[3] We use the concept of *contamination* to refer to processes in which actors are afflicted by something in their surroundings or environment. In contamination processes, something may diffuse from one area or source into another. We may think of specific times and places as contaminated by certain events or processes (e.g. war), products (e.g. tobacco, alcohol), policies, values and ideas (e.g. vengeful spirits). We may ask how people are differently situated and how they are susceptible to or protect themselves from contamination. Common to both contagion and contamination processes are the touch aspects of interactions and exchanges between places, people, animals and things. Etymologically, the words 'contagion' and 'contamination' are derived from Latin *contagio*(n), from con- 'together with' and the base of *tangere* 'to touch' (Oxford Dictionary; see also Meinert and Grøn 2020). The concept denotes the communication or transfer of something between persons, between persons and animals, or between persons and their environment through close contact or touch. This aspect is also central in the story of Alfred and how he and his family are touched by the killing of his brother. The idea of touch resonates well with the local, empirical notion of *cen spirits*, to which we will return.

Configuring in this context describes the interplay between different forms of social contagion and contamination and other biosocial, material and institutional processes occurring over time. Configuring describes the forces which together (con)form the figure of something. In our case afflictions caused by violence, which are labelled differently in different situations or contexts. Configuring is dynamic in that problems and diagnoses change according to which actors, institutions, practices and items are involved. We hope these concepts help to preserve a sense of complexity in understanding individual cases by refraining from associating certain symptoms definitively with final explanatory models. Instead, these concepts highlight how varying configurations at different points in time make up different illness situations, which again change over time and enter into different configurations. This perspective calls for a particular epistemology of pragmatism and a critical phenomenology of violence that pays attention to the way violent experiences touch and affect people.

Alfred's Affliction and Therapeutic Path

The Hospital and Biomedicine
When Alfred's affliction gets worse, his family eventually has him admitted to a local hospital in Gulu Town, where he is given pills and injections with tranquillizers. When we meet Alfred, he cannot recall the different kinds of medication apart from chlorpromazine, an anti-psychotic. However, the most common treatment in cases of *apoya* (madness) is to give combinations of valparin and chlorpromazine, as well as injections with fluphenazine for psychotic episodes and amitriptyline for depressive symptoms.

Alfred is in hospital for four months, during which time he eats and drinks very little. For a long period, he only drinks a bit of milk every day, he explains. The medicine makes him weak and he sleeps a lot. However, when he is awake, he is often aggressive and harasses his fellow patients and the staff, which results in higher doses of medication. His father comes to the ward often to help take care of him. But when his grandmother falls ill in the village, Alfred's father needs to stay there for a lengthy period to take care of her; and during this period Alfred's symptoms get worse. He is told that he tried to escape from the psychiatric ward several times, but he has no recollection of these incidents. More medication is prescribed. Eventually Alfred is tied to his bed by the hospital staff because he is violent towards them.

One of Alfred's brothers, Bennet, reports that the doctors said that Alfred was suffering from *tam ma dwong*: he is 'over-thinking', which is roughly equivalent to the English concept of being stressed or worried. In Bennet's understanding of the doctors' explanation, 'over-thinking' can lead to losing one's senses (*wiye obale*) and to memory failure. Bennet is sceptical about this because he does not think Alfred has any reasons for over-thinking: he has a family and children, and he has a job in the field and as a carpenter. Bennet does not think that the over-thinking results from the death of their brother James:

> James was not only Alfred's brother, he was a brother to us all [in the family]. The other siblings and I have thought a lot about James after his death. I still see his face before me often. But we did not turn mad. And these deaths did not just occur in our family. Almost all families in the village have lost someone to the violence, but there is not madness in every home.

According to Bennet, the explanation is more likely to be found in jealousy and witchcraft. He suspects that someone may have been jealous of Alfred for being young and fairly successful. Alfred was also very good at school, Bennet recalls. These things can create jealousy. Perhaps someone in the village or maybe even in the family went to an *ajwaka*, a witchdoctor, and had misfortune cast on Alfred, Bennet speculates.

Several of our interlocutors explain that a public display of empathy in certain situations can 'open one up' to spiritual contamination. One young man talks about his time with the rebels in the bush, when someone showed obvious sympathy with a person who was being beaten severely by placing his hand on his heart (Meinert and Whyte 2017). Showing empathy in this way can 'open someone up' to spiritual contamination (see also Hopwood and Osburn 2008). This notion of being 'open' by showing empathy points towards ideas of 'porous selves' (Luhrmann 2012; Taylor 2007). If you do not show empathy and harden yourself to the world, it may be possible to resist spiritual contamination in some cases, to resist or make yourself immune to the touch of violence. Perhaps Alfred's close emotional connection to his brother made him receptive and vulnerable when he went to the massacre site to retrieve his brother's body. Seeing and touching his brother's dead body with his hands may have affected Alfred intensely, also due to his young age. Their father may have prepared and hardened himself to the scene, so he was less susceptible to the affect of violence. Family members were open to diverse suggestions regarding what could have caused Alfred's problems, but they usually referred to the cause as 'it' or 'these things', thereby keeping their explanations and possibilities for finding solutions open (Meinert and Whyte 2017; Victor and Porter 2017).

In Dialogue with Spirits

When Alfred is discharged from hospital, he returns to his family in the village. He is not well, but the doctors say that they cannot help him any more. He is still on his medication, although the family does not have the funds for expensive psycho-pharmaceuticals, and they do not think the medication is working well enough. Alfred's mother, Beatrice, takes care of him for lengthy periods assisted by a *lumi yat kwaro*, someone who knows how to use traditional herbs for healing. At first Beatrice has to make the long trip into town to purchase the herbs, but eventually she learns how to identify the plants herself and can pick them in the wild. The herbs seem to have a calming effect on Alfred's symptoms, but he does not heal entirely.

After some time, Beatrice decides to seek help elsewhere, so she goes to a traditional healer, an *ajwaka*. Going to a traditional healer is often a secretive affair, since it arouses suspicion among the neighbours. When people tell their families that they are going to a traditional healer, they usually refrain from saying this directly and instead say '*karo woko*', meaning 'I am going [outside]'. An *ajwaka* is different from a *lumi yat kwaro* (herbal expert) because he/she 'works with the spirits', becoming a medium for the spirits, thereby enabling a dialogue with the dead. This is a practice in which answers and causes are searched for, and it extends beyond symptomatic treatment (Whyte 1997). Beatrice goes to several *ajwaki* (pl.), as people often do before they settle on one that they hope can help find a solution. Alfred is taken to one of the *ajwaki* and stays with her for two months. She initially uses herbs to calm the symptoms and eventually she begins a conversation with the spirits about what they will need in compensation to leave Alfred in peace. The spirits disturbing Alfred, the *ajwaka* explains, are spirits of people who died in the war, they are *cen* spirits (see more on *cen* below).

A contamination took place when Alfred went to pick up the body of his brother, the *ajwaka* suggests, and the 'bad death' that Alfred experienced that day has crept into Alfred's life and body and is making him ill. After two months of herbal treatment and the *ajwaka*'s dialogue with the spirits about his condition, Alfred is feeling better. His symptoms are almost gone, and he returns to his family. Alfred's mother did not have the immediate funds to pay the *ajwaka*, but they managed to make the payment by selling large parts of their crops from the last harvest.[4] During times of conflict and encampment in IDP camps, crops were worth even more than today, because of the danger of going into the fields to work. Alfred's sister tells us that the treatment by the *ajwaka* was controversial in the family, mainly because there were parts of the procedure that indicated that the cause of Alfred's illness might be witchcraft. The finger of suspicion pointed towards Alfred's stepmother, his father's new wife, because her own son, James, had died. The idea was that because of her loss she wanted to hurt Alfred, the son of her husband's former wife. These suspicions never turned into explicit accusations, and they seemed to have been forgotten again.

Alfred starts attending a carpenter college in Gulu Town, and is a student here for three years. After finishing his training, he gets a job in town making furniture. Alfred's symptoms have been gone now for several years. He finds a new group of friends and colleagues in town, they start going out a lot, and Alfred starts to drink and smoke. Smoking marijuana is becoming popular in this period among young men in town.

'It' Returns

On New Year's Eve 2001, the brothers are in town together. They are hanging out outside one of the many small shops, listening to music and drinking. As the night passes, Alfred starts to act strangely. He becomes more aggressive and says things that are out of context. His brothers think that he has had too much to drink. Bennet, however, starts to notice a difference. It is not the usual drunken behaviour. Suddenly, Alfred gets up and runs out of the door and out into the street, where he disappears. The brothers are bewildered and start looking for him. They search the dark streets for a while before they see a group of men beating up someone lying down. It's Alfred, who is lying on the ground. The men are kicking and beating him severely. The brothers run over and plead with the men to let him be, he is ill. The brothers drag Alfred off. The next day Alfred cannot remember the incident. By then the brothers know that he is falling ill again, that 'it' has returned.

The family cannot afford to go back to the traditional healer, so a family meeting is held to find a solution. The family decides that it may be time to turn to the local Pentecostal Church for help and see if they can offer a viable solution for Alfred's condition. Pentecostal churches have been on the rise throughout Uganda since the 1980s (Gusman 2009), and since the end of the war in northern Uganda they seem to be on the rise in this region too. Stephen, one of Alfred's clan brothers, had positive experiences with the local Pentecostal Church and was pushing for this solution, Bennet told us. Stephen encouraged Alfred to turn to the Pentecostal Church for help, and he eventually accepted the suggestion.

Restructuring Life within the Church Community

The local pastor got the congregants together to pray for Alfred. It must be the work of the Devil, he told the family, and prayers were needed. In northern Uganda, explanations that refer to the Devil (*Catan*) are quite different from those referring to spirits. The Devil does not call for dialogue in the way that spirits do. Spirits will often be more personal, have a relation to the family in some way, and will request an animal sacrifice in return for leaving the person alone; whereas the Devil is not to be reasoned with, and must be shunned and driven away. In these cases, people who are born-again Christians (*balokole*) will say that only strong prayer or exorcism helps (Meyer 1999). In other words, there are different ways of configuring violence and affliction.

Before Alfred's treatment in the church, the congregants tell him that to become properly healed he will need to change his life. He 'must accept Jesus Christ as his personal saviour'. He must stop drinking and smoking, there must be no extra-marital sex, he must work hard, go to church gatherings and read the Bible and pray on a daily basis. Alfred agrees to this, thereby accepting a complete restructuring of his daily life. The healing procedure begins with praying and fasting. Alfred goes to the church building in the small village. He stays there for three days with a group of devoted congregants without eating or drinking, only praying. After this initiation, Alfred goes to church every day. At first, he is given small chores: working on the roof of the church with his brethren, going to dig in the field, and using his carpentry skills to repair the broken furniture for the church building. One of the aspects of healing according to the church is that it requires a prolonged change in life, walking a narrow path without wandering astray.

The congregants meet several times a week to pray, and here they pray for Alfred and his illness. After the church ceremony, the pastor and his assistants counsel people. Counselling (*nywako tam*[3]) usually concerns the good and evil forces in the world and how one can stay in the path of God and stay away from sin. Alfred attends all of these activities and starts praying several times a day. He prays when he gets up in the morning, before eating, before work, after work, before dinner and before going to bed. According to Alfred, this started to help him and his symptoms slowly disappear again. In 2019, Alfred is still an active member of the Pentecostal Church.

The fact that Alfred ended up finding stability and healing in the Pentecostal Church is not necessarily an argument in favour of the specific Christian content of the church activities. Instead, we would emphasize the importance of the kind of structure that life in this kind of community involves. The planning and structuring of daily activities are often recommended for people suffering from PTSD (Zoellner, Sacks and Foa 2001).

These dynamics of affliction and recovery can be understood as kinds of social contagion and contamination within changing configurations. When we ask Alfred himself, he simply says that 'you can fall ill from all kinds of things – but now I am well again'. He does not seem particularly interested in speculating about causes. When we interviewed Alfred again in 2019, and asked him to reflect on his story, he said that the prayer and fasting had helped him recover. He expressed regret about the money spent on the traditional healer, but thought that the medication he received in the hospital helped him sleep during hard times and prevented him from becoming violent towards others while he was in hospital. In other words, the medicine stopped the touch of violence from spreading, but was not, according to Alfred, what finally made him well.

We attempt to stick with Alfred's perspective in some sense by refraining from presenting explanations based on discrete idioms like 'trauma' or '*cen* spirits', and observing instead what people do and how they manage their affliction in daily life. The advantage of this approach is that it makes it possible to show how different afflictions are configured and formed in response to different epistemologies of healing. These are not static and discrete systems of interpretation and healing. On the contrary, notions of spirits, trauma and the Devil are all pragmatic concepts applied in specific situations to give a direction to action, which in turn changes and transforms the afflictions.

The events leading to Alfred's illness – the death of his brother James, the hospitalization, the family's financial situation, the traditional healers and church community – are all part of the changing configurations that make up his story. We argue that his illness and path towards recovery cannot be reduced or explained by any one of these alone. These different contexts of healing all influence each other, they all become aspects of the changing configurations that make up Alfred's course and experience of illness. Viewing the story through this lens makes it possible to show what people do from situation to situation and how these actions change, without linking the explanation inextricably to idioms of 'spirits' or 'trauma'. Whenever Alfred moves into a new treatment context, new aspects are brought into focus and new authorities are put in place. New configurations are created. In the following we focus on two main notions which are widespread in the Acholi region at present: the traditional notion of *cen*, and the biomedical notion of trauma.

Cen and Trauma: Paths of Contamination and Practices of Treatment

Two central – and often overlapping and intertwined – notions of affliction in northern Uganda are the local concept of *cen* and the global psychological concept of trauma. Both of these are ways to express the influence or touch of violence. Both notions spread as explanatory categories and configure with other idioms, actors, institutions and materialities, leading to a variety of treatment practices. In the following we show how these notions are used, how they become relevant in people's lives, and how they take part in larger configurations in the Acholi region and global discourses.

Cen: When 'Bad Death' Contaminates

In the literature, *cen* is predominantly described as a spiritual problem or contamination connected to 'bad death'. If you are involved in killing, or find yourself in areas where massacres have taken place, or treat dead bodies in an undignified way, you can be spiritually contaminated (Meinert and Whyte 2017; Victor and Porter 2017). The concept can be found in the literature on northern Uganda at least as far back as the writing of the Verona Fathers, who came to the Acholi region as missionaries in 1913. In his notes on the Acholi language, Father Crazzolara describes *cen* as 'a departed spirit, vengefully disposed' (Crazzolara [1933] 1938: 199). Versions of this can be found in all Nilotic languages (p'Bitek 1971). E.E. Evans-Pritchard also wrote about *cen* (*cien*) among the Nuer, a neighbouring ethnic group in Sudan, where 'it means the vengeance, generally producing sickness or other misfortune ending in death, taken by an aggrieved ghost on the living, and in its verbal form the taking of such vengeance' (Evans-Pritchard 1949: 291). *Cen* is thus characterized by a broad spectrum of expressions: being haunted by the dead, wandering alone in the bush, sleeping in the bush, becoming distracted, ears ringing, loss of wits, child deaths and other misfortunes. Many people also emphasize that *cen* is something that can be contagious from person to person – for example, it can be generated by the killing and torture of people in the bush and can then be brought back to the village, where it will spread in a contagious manner. But you can also be contaminated by *cen* when you walk through an area where killing has taken place. In these cases, opportunities for action may also focus on areas and not people. The cleansing ritual *moyo piny* results in the cleansing of an area, as opposed to *moyo kum*, which is the cleansing of a person or body.

Configuring *cen* today plays into global imaginaries. As one informant told us, when we asked for his views on *cen*: '*Cen* is what is happening in Syria [the killing of civilians in 2017], *cen* is all kinds of sinful behaviour, it is also the dead coming back and disturbing people, it is all of these things'. Technology and materiality also play into the evolving picture. When people were killed with spears in a local conflict in the past, the conflicting parties could always see who had initiated the action and who would bear the responsibility (Hutchinson 1996: 107). However, developments in weapons technology and the introduction of landmines and machine guns have created new paths of contamination and new configurations. Besides generating more dead bodies, the new weapon technologies can hide the fact of who the killer is, because people can be killed from great distances without the killer being identified.

Trauma: The Spread of a Global Term

The imaginary of trauma has travelled since the end of the Vietnam War to all corners of the world in a manner that has made experts talk of 'an empire of trauma' (Fassin and Rechtman 2009). The notion of trauma has also reached northern Uganda in several versions. One version is the distinct, monolithic category of post-traumatic stress disorder (PTSD) based on diagnostic criteria contained in the American Psychological Organization's DSM manual. This distinct understanding of trauma is widespread in hospitals and among psychotherapeutically oriented NGOs (Williams 2020). The notion of trauma in everyday discourse, on the other hand, has a life of its own and is used about all kinds of maladies and misfortunes (Williams 2021).

The history of the concept of trauma in northern Uganda can be traced back to the HIV/AIDS programmes in the 1990s (Whyte in Vorhölter 2019). An interlocutor from the village told us that he first heard of 'trauma' when he worked for one of the foreign NGOs working with HIV/AIDS treatment. Here it became known that a positive HIV diagnosis 'could cause trauma in people'. The NGO staff were therefore trained in psychotherapeutic counselling. In this way the notion of counselling became connected to the notion of trauma, as it did elsewhere in Uganda (Whyte et al. 2013).

Most important for the spread of notions of trauma and psychotherapeutic selves in northern Uganda was the establishment of reception centres in the 1990s. These centres were established in order to receive homecoming abductees or soldiers who had been with the LRA in the bush. A very large number of children and young people used these reception centres during the years of conflict.[6] In the centres there was an emphasis on psychological trauma and the importance of psychological counselling (Verma 2012). Several reception centres collaborated with NGOs which could help people after they left the centres. In northern Uganda today there are still NGOs working explicitly with psychological trauma therapy, with many providing psychosocial interventions or activities (Torre 2019; Vorhölter 2019). Psychoeducation is part of these interventions and is one of the clearest examples of how specific notions of the mind and trauma from the Global North are introduced in the region (Williams 2020).

The Spread of Violence and Search for Relief

Interpreting these phenomena – as forms of touch by a violent history and specific events – provides a different lens for understanding the expanding phenomena of trauma and *cen* spirits.

What we see in Alfred's story and in the homes of families trying to help their relatives suffering from mental illness in a variety of ways is not a well-established empire of trauma relief that is spreading. The notion of trauma has been widely appropriated and is often used in a variety of ways to express different kinds of conditions which collapse a series of local expressions into the term 'trauma' (Williams 2021); but the options for and uptake of actual trauma relief are scarce. The potential for an empire of trauma relief may be present, but it lacks a functioning infrastructure (Meinert and Whyte 2020). The treatment of PTSD seems helpful for some, but the efforts of NGOs are not sufficient given the extent of the mental health problems in northern Uganda. The diagnosis and treatment of PTSD are largely in the hands of these NGOs. PTSD is far less visible in government health facilities, even in the public facility that has a mental health clinic run by psychiatric nurses and clinical officers. Yet the public health system is more widely available and is also a constant presence, whereas NGO projects come and go.

As we saw earlier, despite his experiences of violence and death, Alfred does not think of himself as traumatized or haunted by *cen* spirits. He is not very interested in what 'it' was and what caused it. He is not searching for psychological or other explanations, he is searching for relief and has found that his work routines and prayer regime help.

Epistemologies of *Cen* and Trauma

The relationship between the imaginaries surrounding *cen* and trauma is complex. One initial argument for looking at the two together is that they both seem to express very similar symptomatologies. Alfred's symptoms of aggression, nightmares, memory loss and visions, which seem to be connected to past experiences of violence, can perhaps be classified as both *cen* and trauma. There is also a similar temporality to these symptoms, which can be both defined and understood based on prior experiences of violence (Williams and Meinert 2020). In different ways, they are also combined for people in everyday life. Some of the psychiatric nurses we interviewed (who had been trained to use psychiatric vocabulary) would describe the relationship as 'the spirits can give you PTSD, and in that case, you need medicine and counselling for the PTSD and prayers against the spirits'. During another interview a retired psychiatrist told us that '*cen* and other traditional ideas' were simply local words for trauma, and that traditional rituals were a kind of mental illness treatment (although according to the psychiatrist, they were inferior to medicine and counselling), thereby collapsing the traditional world of spirits into a clinical biomedical interpretation.[7] Within the many Pentecostal churches, people suffering from 'these things' are also sometimes referred to as 'trauma persons', and it is very common here to combine biomedicine with prayers as the safest path towards recovery. Time and resources are also essential elements in these configurations. As mentioned above, cleansing rituals are increasingly expensive and village families with an average income can only afford them if they save up for a long time. Psycho-pharmaceuticals are also very expensive and are therefore often taken ad hoc based not necessarily on prescriptions, but on the income of the month and whatever is in stock at the pharmacy or in the hospital. Temporal dimensions are also essential here. For instance, some of the NGOs administer psychotherapeutic treatments which normally involve ten to twelve one-hour sessions, after which the client is expected to be on a steady path towards recovery. But the path of recovery in the church community is a lifelong project requiring the client to maintain a righteous lifestyle through a daily prayer regime and weekly rituals with the other congregants.

Our contribution here contains several elements. By discussing Alfred's problems as an extended case, we have shown the configuration of affliction in a life, family and situation over time. We have described the meagre but multiple treatment options for mental illness in northern Uganda after the war, and the pragmatism that people use in finding solutions to these problems. Here action and alleviation are central, rather than final explanations and categorizations of the origin and cause of problems (Meinert and Whyte 2017; Victor and Porter 2017; Williams 2019). We have attempted to show not simply that people combine the options in a variety of ways, but that the very expression of these illnesses transforms and changes when they are configured through different paths of recovery and within different epistemological approaches. It is not simply a market of healing with churches, NGOs, hospitals and traditional healers offering their services; these institutions tap into each other in a myriad of ways as people travel through them in search of relief from their disorders. The symptomatic expressions are changed and transformed as they become practices within new contexts, labelled anew and treated as *cen*, as trauma or as demonic intervention. This speaks to current debates not only about post-conflict dynamics in northern Uganda and elsewhere, but also to theoretical and conceptual debates about how to conceptualize mental illness as something dynamic and transforming (Kirmayer, Lemelson and Cummings 2015; Luhrmann and Marrow 2016), as well as debates about what role trauma should have in anthropological analysis more generally (Argenti 2016; Robbins 2013). With the concept of configuration, we have highlighted that mental illness, or problems with trauma and spirits, exist and spread as part of changing configurations. The increase of violence as part of war was the most significant changing factor for the spread of trauma and spirit afflictions in northern Uganda. The changes in discourse, institutions and options for treatment were important, but secondary, to the configuration of the spread of these afflictions. The configuration analysis of how mental afflictions spread with a point of departure in notions of touch may be a conceptual addition to related literature, which has explored mental illness through concepts such as embodiment (Csordas and Jenkins 2018, social defeat (Luhrmann and Marrow 2016) and ecosocial approaches (Kirmayer, Lemelson and Cummings 2015). We hope that Alfred's case has demonstrated not just that mental illness, trauma or problems with spirits are changing phenomena, but furthermore how they spread through different kinds of touch: through contagion and contamination in and between people, places, institutions and practices. The way Alfred is touched by the experience of violence, by his brother James's dead body, by the psychotropic medication in the hospital and by the prayer in church, indicates the way in which contagious and contaminating elements from a legacy of violence can con-figure – give figure to – afflictions of spirits and trauma. A legacy that transforms as it moves through families and generations and touches people on its way.

Acknowledgements

We are grateful to Alfred and his family, as well as other interlocutors in northern Uganda, for sharing their experiences and views and letting us get a glimpse into their lifeworlds. Many thanks go to our good colleagues at Gulu University, who have hosted our studies and provided their insights. We thank the AU Research Foundation for funding EPICENTER and the work that preceded this edited book. We are grateful to the three anonymous reviewers for their helpful comments and suggestions for the chapter.

The case described in this chapter has been translated from the article in Danish: Williams, L.H., and Meinert, L. (2017). 'Traumer og Ånder efter Krig i Uganda: Konfigurationer af Vold og Behandling', *Tidsskrift for Forskning i Sygdom og Samfund*, 14(26). Permission has been granted by the journal *Tidsskrift for Forskning i Sygdom og Samfund*.

Lars Williams
PhD, Aarhus University, Denmark
Visiting Fellow, London School of Economics and Political Science, UK

Lotte Meinert
Professor, Department of Anthropology
Aarhus University, Denmark

Notes

1. All interlocutors and relatives have been given pseudonyms to ensure anonymity.
2. We situate ourselves close to the experience-oriented anthropological tradition, in which single interlocutors, families and particular contexts play a central part (Das 2015; Good 1993; Mattingly 2014).
3. Hartmut Rosa's (2019) notion of resonance and the human capacity for being touched, moved and marked describes mainly the positive side of being affected by a relationship to the world. Here we focus on the darker and fragile side of this relationship.
4. The cost of cleansing rituals in northern Uganda rose significantly after the end of the war, and this was often one of the most expensive types of healing. This may also be part of the reason why so many people started to seek help in the churches, where healing procedures are cheap or even free.
5. Literally meaning 'sharing thoughts'.
6. It has been hard to determine how many. According to Allen and Schomerus (2006), the number varies a good deal from year to year (more than four thousand people in 2003 and down to around six hundred in 2005).
7. This is similar to what Abramowitz (2010) has described in Liberia with the local notion of open mole.

References

Abramowitz, S.A. 2010. 'Trauma and Humanitarian Translation in Liberia: The Tale of Open Mole', *Culture, Medicine, and Psychiatry* 34(2), 353–79.

Allen, T., and M. Schomerus. 2006. 'A Hard Homecoming: Lessons Learned from the Reception Center Process in Northern Uganda', *Washington, DC: Management Systems International* 62(7).

Amone-P'Olak, K., S.B. Dokkedahl and A. Elklit. 2017. 'Post-Traumatic Stress Disorder among Child Perpetrators and Victims of Violence from the Northern Uganda Civil War: Findings from the WAYS Study', *Journal of Psychology in Africa* 27(3): 235–42.

Argenti, N. 2016. 'Laughter without Borders: Embodied Memory, and Pan-Humanism in a Post-Traumatic Age', in V. Broch-Due and B.E. Bertelsen (eds), *Violent Reverberations*. London: Palgrave Macmillan, pp. 241–68.

Crazzolara, J.P. [1933] 1938. *Outlines of a Nuer Grammar*. Vienna: Verlag der Internationalen Zeitschrift.

Csordas, T.J., and J.H. Jenkins. 2018. 'Living with a Thousand Cuts: Self-Cutting, Agency, and Mental Illness among Adolescents', *Ethos* 46(2), 206–29.

Das, V. 2015. *Affliction: Health, Disease, Poverty*. New York: Fordham University Press.

Dolan, C. 2008. *Social Torture: The Case of Northern Uganda, 1986–2006*. New York: Berghahn Books.

Evans-Pritchard, E.E. 1949. 'Nuer Curses and Ghostly Vengeance', *Africa* 19(4): 288–92.

——— . 1965. *Theories of Primitive Religion*. Oxford: Clarendon Press.

Fassin, D., and R. Rechtman. 2009. *The Empire of Trauma: An Inquiry into the Condition of Victimhood*. Princeton, NJ: Princeton University Press.

Gluckman, M. 1961. 'Ethnographic Data in British Social Anthropology', *The Sociological Review* 9(1): 5–17.

Good, B.J. 1993. *Medicine, Rationality and Experience: An Anthropological Perspective*. Cambridge: Cambridge University Press.

Gusman, A. 2009. 'HIV/AIDS, Pentecostal churches, and the "Joseph Generation" in Uganda', *Africa Today* 56(1), 67–86.

Hopwood, J., and C. Osburn. 2008. *Sharing the Burden of the Past: Peer Support and Self Help amongst Former Lord's Resistance Army Youth*. Gulu: The Justice and Reconciliation Project, Quaker Peace and Social Witness.

Hutchinson, S.E. 1996. *Nuer Dilemmas: Coping with Money, War, and the State*. Oakland: University of California Press.

Kirmayer, L.J., R. Lemelson and C.A. Cummings (eds). 2015. *Re-Visioning Psychiatry: Cultural Phenomenology, Critical Neuroscience, and Global Mental Health*. Cambridge: Cambridge University Press.

Luhrmann, T.M. 2012. *When God Talks Back: Understanding the American Evangelical Relationship with God*. New York: Vintage.

Luhrmann, T.M., and J. Marrow (eds). 2016. *Our Most Troubling Madness: Case Studies in Schizophrenia across Cultures*. Oakland: University of California Press.

Mattingly, C. 2014. *Moral Laboratories: Family Peril and the Struggle for a Good Life*. Oakland: University of California Press.

Meinert, L. 2015. 'Tricky Trust: Distrust as a Point of Departure and Trust as a Social Achievement in Uganda', in S. Liisberg, E.O. Pedersen and A.L. Dalsgård (eds), *Anthropology and Philosophy: Dialogues on Trust and Hope*. New York: Berghahn Books, pp. 118–36.

Meinert, L., and L. Grøn 2020. ' "It Runs in the Family": Exploring Contagious Kinship Connections', *Ethnos* 85(4), 581–94.

Meinert, L., and S.R. Whyte. 2017. '"These Things Continue": Violence as Contamination in Everyday Life after War in Northern Uganda', *Ethos* 45(2): 271–86.

——— . 2020. 'Legacies of Violence: The Communicability of Spirits and Trauma in Northern Uganda', in J. Seeberg, A. Roepstorff and L. Meinert (eds), *Biosocial Worlds: Anthropology of Health Environments beyond Determinism*. London: UCL Press, pp. 168–90.

Meinert, L., J.A. Obika and S.R. Whyte. 2014. 'Crafting Forgiveness Accounts after War: Editing for Effect in Northern Uganda', *Anthropology Today* 30: 10–14.

Meyer, B. 1999. *Translating the Devil: Religion and Modernity among the Ewe in Ghana*. Edinburgh: Edinburgh University Press.

Oboke, H., S.R. Whyte. 2020. 'Anger and Bitter Hearts: The Spread of Suicide in Northern Ugandan Families', *Ethnos* 85(4), 612–28.

p'Bitek, O. 1971. *Religion of the Central Luo*. Nairobi: Kenya Literature Bureau.

Robbins, J. 2004. 'The Globalization of Pentecostal and Charismatic Christianity', *Annual Review of Anthropology* 33: 117–43.

——. 2013. 'Beyond the Suffering Subject: Toward an Anthropology of the Good', *Journal of the Royal Anthropological Institute* 19(3): 447–62.

Rosa, H. 2019. *Resonance: A Sociology of Our Relationship to the World*. Hoboken, NJ: John Wiley & Sons.

Rose, N. 1990. *Governing the Soul: The Shaping of the Private Self*. London: Routledge.

Rosenberg, C.E. 1992. *Explaining Epidemics and other Studies in the History of Medicine*. New York: Cambridge University Press.

Schiltz, J., and K. Büscher. 2018. 'Brokering Research with War-Affected People: The Tense Relationship between Opportunities and Ethics', *Ethnography* 19(1): 124–46.

Seeberg, J., and L. Meinert. 2015. 'Can Epidemics be Noncommunicable? Reflections on the Spread of Noncommunicable Diseases', *Medicine Anthropological Theory* 2(2): 54–71.

Taylor, C. 2007. *A Secular Age*. Cambridge, MA: Harvard University Press.

Torre, C. 2019. 'Psychosocial Support (PSS) in War-Affected Countries: A Literature Review', Politics of Return Working Paper, no. 3. London: London School of Economics.

Van Velsen, J. 2017. 'The Extended-Case Method and Situational Analysis', in A.L. Epstein (ed.), *The Craft of Social Anthropology*. London: Routledge, pp. 129–50.

Verma, C.L. 2012. 'Truths Out of Place: Homecoming, Intervention, and Story-Making in War-Torn Northern Uganda', *Children's Geographies* 10: 441–55. https://doi.org/10.1080/14.

Victor, L., and H. Porter. 2017. 'Dirty Things: Spiritual Pollution and Life after the Lord's Resistance Army', *Journal of Eastern African Studies* 11(4): 590–608.

Vorhölter, J. 2019. 'Struggling to Be a "Happy Self"? Psychotherapy and the Medicalization of Unhappiness in Uganda', *Current Anthropology: A World Journal of the Sciences of Man* 2: 194–223.

Whyte, S.R. 1997. *Questioning Misfortune: The Pragmatics of Uncertainty in Eastern Uganda*. Cambridge: Cambridge University Press.

Whyte, S.R., et al. 2013. 'Remaining Internally Displaced: Missing Links to Human Security in Northern Uganda', *Journal of Refugee Studies* 26(2): 283–301.

Williams, L.H. 2019. 'In Search of a Stable World: Contamination of Spirits and Mental Disorder in Post-Conflict Northern Uganda', Ph.D. dissertation. Aarhus: Aarhus University.

———. 2020. 'Training Theories of Mind in Post-Conflict Northern Uganda', *Medical Anthropology* 40(2): 196–207. doi:10.1080/01459740.2020.1802722.

———. 2021. 'Negotiating Languages of Suffering in Northern Uganda', *Qualitative Studies* 6(1): 159–82.

Williams, L.H., and L. Meinert. 2017. 'Traumer og Ånder efter Krig i Uganda: Konfigurationer af Vold og Behandling', *Tidsskrift for Forskning i Sygdom og Samfund* 14(26): 63–88.

———. 2020. 'Repetition Work: Healing Spirits and Trauma in the Churches of Northern Uganda', in M. Flaherty, L. Dalsgaard and L. Meinert (eds), *Time Work: Studies of Temporal Agency*. New York: Berghahn Books, pp. 31–49.

Zoellner, L.A., M.B. Sacks and E.B. Foa. 2001. 'Stability of Emotions for Traumatic Memories in Acute and Chronic PTSD', *Behaviour Research and Therapy* 39(6): 697–711.

Chapter 7
'These Spirit Attacks Are Like an Epidemic'
Spirit Possession as Affective Contagion in Niger

Adeline Masquelier, Abouzeidi Maidouka Dillé and Ly Amadou H. Belko

> Society is imitation and imitation is a kind of somnambulism.
>
> —Gabriel Tarde, *The Laws of Imitation*

> The potential stored in ordinary things is a network of transfers and relays. Fleeting and amorphous, it lives as a residue or resonance in an emergent assemblage of disparate forms and realms of life. Yet it can be as palpable as a physical trace.
>
> —Kathleen Stewart, *Ordinary Affects*

On 18 May 2009 a number of schoolgirls participating in an athletic exercise in Niamey, Niger's capital, allegedly succumbed to 'hysteria' following the sudden intrusion of a *génie tchatcheur* (chatty demon) in their midst. Reports of the incident sent chills across the city. Yet most people were not exactly surprised. Rumours had it the infamous spirit possessed scantily dressed adolescent girls. In fact, a similar outbreak had occurred days earlier at a nearby school, causing great havoc and forcing local authorities to close the establishment momentarily. A witness recalled how panic had swept through the school after a girl suddenly darted across the courtyard, shrieking and flailing her arms. Her screams set off

'These Spirit Attacks Are Like an Epidemic'

other female students, and in a matter of minutes, half a dozen girls were jumping in the air and running in all directions, seemingly possessed by invisible forces.[1] One of them had a wild look in her eyes; she was saying strange things. When a couple of teachers tried to restrain her, she insulted them in a deep, gruff voice. Classes were suspended and alerted parents soon turned up at the school to collect their children. Meanwhile four of the afflicted girls were brought to the hospital for diagnosis and treatment. The next day the school reopened and classes were held without further disruptions. Some parents nevertheless confessed to being worried about their daughters' safety since no ritual had been performed to rid the establishment of the demonic presence. Meanwhile nearly everyone in the neighbourhood had something to say about the proliferation of spiritual attacks in educational settings.

The past two decades or so have witnessed a remarkable number of episodes of 'mass hysteria' in secondary schools across Niger (Masquelier 2020). In classrooms, on playgrounds, or during gym sessions adolescent girls (and more rarely young female teachers) are reportedly possessed by violent, rash, vindictive jinn (in Hausa *aljanu*; masculine singular *aljani*; feminine singular *aljana*) claiming to have been wronged in a (not so) distant past.[2] Possession is often contagious. Minutes after a girl shows signs of being overtaken by a spirit, others in her vicinity will start screeching, moaning, jumping or thrashing around, and before long, half the classroom has succumbed to possession. In 2006 a television crew captured an outbreak of mass possession involving as many as fifty schoolgirls; the incident was later broadcast on Télé Sahel, Niger's primary television channel. The mayhem that ensued compelled local authorities to close the school until religious specialists could cleanse it of evil influences. Possession episodes – often characterized as spiritual attacks – typically elicit great alarm. Paradoxically, they have become frequent enough that some teachers now see them as an inevitable dimension of school life – an 'inconvenience' they just have to put up with.[3] Even so, the girls' screams and disorderly behaviour can cause significant commotion, forcing local authorities to momentarily close the school. Teachers have complained to us that owing to the number of class days 'lost to the spirits', they rarely complete the academic curriculum on schedule; they are often forced to rush through the programme of study or skip parts of it.[4]

Aside from momentarily disrupting the tempo of school life, the possession of adolescent schoolgirls opens up a critical space for articulating the past as 'unfinished business'. When spiritual healers perform exorcisms to rid the victims of their spiritual tormentors, a story emerges that typically goes something like this: some time ago people cut down trees to make room for a new school or expand an existing one. The spirits who lived in these trees were displaced. They now reportedly haunt the very building whose erection contributed to their displacement. Their lingering presence among schoolchildren is a source of great concern for parents and teachers, not to mention the children themselves.

At another level, the spirits' eviction points to a broader history of iconoclasm aimed at purifying Islam from unwarranted innovations (*bidi'a* in Hausa). Niger, an overwhelmingly Muslim country, has witnessed several waves of religious fervour that resulted in the progressive erasure of spirit-centred practices in the past century. Spirit possession ceremonies, once a central dimension of health-seeking practices and a popular form of entertainment as well as a wellspring of political resistance, became vilified as a source of immorality and an index of backwardness.[5] Muslim preachers now describe spirits in their sermons as malevolent creatures who lure humans away from the rightful path. In no circumstances should they be invited to possess humans. Nor should they be placated through offerings of any kind (for only Qur'anic verses should be used to protect oneself against spirits or chase them away). In the late 1980s, young men increasingly refused to marry girls who attended possession ceremonies and husbands divorced women who 'had spirits'. Following the emergence of Izala,[6] a reformist Muslim movement that sought to reassert the role of Islam in public and private life (Niandou-Souley and Alzouma 1996), Muslim preachers actively discouraged exorcisms, arguing that any kind of dealing with jinn was un-Islamic: *aljanu* were Satan's servants and Muslims should not interact with them, not even to get rid of them. It has since become commonplace for Muslim religious leaders to denounce spirit-based therapeutics as well as amulets and other Qur'an-based medicines and rely strictly on biomedicine (while putting their faith in God). In the process, many people (at least officially) turned their backs on the spirits to affirm their modernity and moral uprightness.

In highlighting the boundaries of the moral order, Izala recast the definition of virtuous femininity in contrast to Western models of womanhood perceived as a symbol of decadence and depravity (Masquelier 2009). Against the backdrop of moralizing discourses that brought increased scrutiny to women as embodiments of virtue, the possession of schoolgirls was linked to female dissipation and immodesty. Brash girls who did not veil invited spirits to possess them, many reformist Muslim preachers proclaimed in their sermons, inferring that the girls' improper body coverage – and the lack of virtue it implied – was what attracted the spirits to them (some spirits, including *génies tchatcheurs*, reportedly 'fall in love' with humans and seduce them).[7] Today Muslim preachers of all persuasions routinely disparage female adolescents whose bare heads and revealing clothes mark them as bearers of Western contamination.[8] Capitalizing on the panic elicited by the spectacle of schoolgirls in the throes of possession, they evoke moral decline and urge women and girls to veil and follow the Qur'an's teaching to prevent further spiritual attacks. Meanwhile the efflorescence of spiritual attacks in secondary schools has been a financial boon for religious specialists claiming expertise in the art of *rukiyya* (exorcism).

Not everyone in Niger subscribes to the thesis that schools are haunted by spirits, however. School administrators who must handle the crises are often reluctant to give in to 'superstition', relying instead on the diagnosis of physicians who categorize trance as a conversion disorder, a psychosomatic syndrome whose origin lies in the patient's inability to deal with some prior trauma or conflict. They typically reject parental requests that ritual specialists be hired to cleanse the schools of toxic spiritual influences, fearful such interventions could be a drain on their already modest budgets. Occasionally, they capitulate to pressure, especially when funding from school management committees and local government is available. Government officials are similarly inclined to describe possession episodes as collective forms of hysteria requiring psychiatric treatment. Alternatively, they invoke stress or epilepsy and insist that parents bring their afflicted daughters to the hospital.

One might argue that diagnostics of mass hysteria sit jaggedly alongside chronicles of ecological loss and allegations of female corruption and immodesty. Yet what emerges from the various testimonies about these phenomena that we have collected is a sense that something is afflicting schoolgirls on a massive level. Not only can the affliction 'contaminate' an entire classroom in a matter of minutes, but it also travels from one school to another. The reports of what happens to the afflicted girls are strikingly similar regardless of which school they attend. To be sure, details occasionally surface that are specific to one of the victims, such as a spirit falling in love with a pretty girl and tormenting her out of possessiveness. A pattern nevertheless emerges from these testimonies, which points to the contagious nature of the schoolgirls' affliction. Like an epidemic, it comes without warning, spreads across an entire school (or select classrooms), and later fades away.

Rather than drawing on anthropological models that frame spirit possession as individual resistance, the somatization of unconscious desire, or a kind of localizing discourse for dealing with conflict (Masquelier 2018; Ong 1988; Sharp 1990), in this chapter we attend to the relational dimensions of the girls' affliction through the analytical prism of contagion. By taking spirit possession to be a form of 'circulating affliction' (Seale-Feldman 2019: 312), we address the problem of schoolgirls' susceptibility, that is, their openness and impressionability, to others. Inspired by the incipient anthropology of intangibles (Espírito Santo and Blanes 2014), we consider the lives of spirits by tracing the symptoms and effects they produce in our interlocutors' own lives. In what follows, we discuss the rash of spiritual attacks occurring in Nigerien schools by drawing on the model of contagion elaborated by Gabriel Tarde to account for the rapid spread of ideas, fashions, technologies and crimes across a population. Diagnosing the possession of schoolgirls as 'hysteria' or 'conversion disorder', whereby a psychological experience is converted into bodily affliction, does not account for how ideas and emotions spread and 'infect' certain people. Through a focus on imitation – by which he meant the ability to affect and be affected, consciously and unconsciously, by others – Tarde put the accent on the extraordinary 'magnetic' power people can exert over each other in their interactions. Following Tarde, we tentatively argue that the mass possession of Nigerien schoolgirls instantiates how persons incorporate others into themselves and are themselves embodied in others, a process that can be described as a contagion without contact. The subsequent analysis is primarily informed by fieldwork conducted in the *département* of Dogondoutchi in

2018, though it also draws on three decades of research by Adeline Masquelier in Niger, most of it focused on spirit possession and other forms of religious engagement.

From Somatization to Contagion

When stricken schoolgirls are brought to the hospital, psychiatrists or psychosocial counsellors (if they are available) will likely diagnose them with 'conversion disorder'. Stories of vindictive spirits are set aside. They are incommensurable with medical models based on a mind/body split, in which unacknowledged mental suffering finds expression in physical ailments. Interviewed for a recently published article on 'the scientific explanations' for the mass possession of schoolgirls, Nigerien psychologist Zourkaleini Issa Maiga observed that conversion disorder was a psychiatric illness whose symptoms were 'a response to something in the patient's life' (Oumar 2019). The symptoms, he stressed, frequently arose among girls who experienced 'the loss of their parents, physical or psychological abuse, rape and sexual harassment, academic struggles, deceptions' (ibid.). While conversion disorder could afflict girls as young as seven, the symptoms did not typically develop until age fourteen, when girls were in the throes of puberty. The malady, Dr Maiga noted, was known in the educational environment under the appellation of *génies tchatcheurs*.

One may infer from Dr Maiga's testimony that the possession of schoolgirls in Niger is a focus of psychosocial interventions. In reality, few afflicted girls have access to psychiatric services.[9] Indeed, the vast majority of Nigeriens are unfamiliar with psychosocial diagnoses. Parents seeking relief for what ails their daughters frequently turn to religious specialists who rely on the Qur'an, herbs or mediumistic powers to heal the sick. Rather than locating the source of the malady in an unresolved trauma or conflict that 'speaks' through the body, as psychiatrists do, these religious specialists attribute the problem to *aljanu* avenging themselves for slights they previously experienced. They cure their patients by expelling the spiteful creatures that are tormenting them.[10] At the demands of parents, they may also cleanse the school of demonic influences. Whether they attend to possessed individuals, haunted buildings or both, the curative practices they perform share with epidemiology a concern with limiting exposure to the sources of contagion by breaking the chain of transmission and neutralizing the infectious agent. The focus of their intervention is the communicability (i.e. transmission) *between* people rather than *within* individuals, as psychiatric models (based on the mind/body split) would have it.

Such transmission is most effectively captured through the language of affect and attunement, which is why we speak of contagion – a process in which the behaviour of one person inspires (or is copied by) other persons. But that is not all. When people speak of cleansing a school of its sinister occupants, the presence of the spirits is seen as a form of contamination, a noxious influence that is part of the setting. Writing on *cen*, the Acholi spirits of the dead who have died a violent death in Uganda, Lotte Meinert and Susan Reynolds Whyte observe that *cen* affliction is conceptualized as contamination rather than contagion. Whereas contagion refers to a process of transmission by means of touch, contamination 'happens in an environment, sometimes as a process of seeping through layers (of soils, souls, and socialities)' (Meinert and Whyte 2017: 284). In Niger, too, haunted schools are perceived as contaminated buildings in which the violence of the past lives as both residue and resonance 'in an emergent assemblage of disparate forms and realms of life' (Stewart 2007: 21).

It is worth noting that while many people hold *aljanu* responsible for the chaos erupting in schools, some suspect that manipulation is at play, engineered by the 'victims' themselves. 'Sometimes it feels like the girls do it for fun. I once slapped a girl who was coming at me like mad. She started coughing and [the trance] was over. Since then, nothing. The spirits are leaving her alone, which means perhaps that she did it on purpose, that one time', a former student volunteered. Masquelier was told that after the director of a professional school in Niamey threatened to expel 'all the girls who screamed', not a single possession incident had been observed in the school. People frequently noted that many spirit attacks occur right before the start of examinations. A friend recalled that baccalaureate athletic examinations were reportedly put off in 2009 in Konni, a town near the Nigerian border, after several girls fell to the ground, twisting and turning before losing consciousness. 'You hand students the questions for the math test. And soon after some girls start screaming or fainting, so the exam is cancelled. This is no coincidence. It's a known fact that girls are not good at science', is how a male university student put it. Implicit in these testimonies is the recognition that girls also command a form of power when they disrupt school activities with their screams, jumps and bodily contortions.

On the basis of reports of exam cancellations and school closures, one might conclude that possession is a form of resistance. Girls who struggle in school find ways to avoid being tested or even to attend school altogether. By disrupting school activities, they express a malaise that finds no other language. Such an interpretation lines up with anthropological models that frame possession as a means through which the dispossessed and the marginalized deal with the challenges of life (Boddy 1989; Masquelier 2001; Ong 1988). In their respective studies of possessed schoolgirls in Nigeria, Madagascar and Kenya, Susan O'Brien (2001), Lesley Sharp (1993) and James Smith (2001) put the accent on the struggles adolescent girls face. According to Sharp (1990: 339), schoolgirls who transitioned from rural to town life in northwest Madagascar 'suffer from the contradictions of a fragmented world'. Through possession they give shape to the chaos inherent in their existence. Dorothy Hodgson (1997) has similarly argued that possession among the Maasai provides a means of embodying the contradictions of Tanzanian modernity. Masquelier (2018) has suggested that the possession of Nigerien schoolgirls offers a critical commentary on the moralization of education in contexts of heightened religiosity. The problem with these interpretations is that they rely on an agentive model of personhood based on Western liberal concepts of autonomy and freedom (Mahmood 2005) while ignoring local etiologies of mass possession. Moreover, the broad resonances between these various cases of youth possession across Africa create something of a problem for the analysis of *aljanu*: there are so many similarities between the interpretive frameworks proposed by the analysts that the concepts they rely on lose their sharpness. It becomes difficult to recover the particularities of the Nigerien experience, submerged as it is by an overdetermined narrative of agency, resistance and somatization.

The alternative means attending to lay people's diagnoses of mass possession. Such diagnoses typically rely on notions of exposure and contagion, thereby shifting the focus from individuality to relationality. In the words of a history and geography teacher who had been teaching at the same school for fifteen years, 'the spirit attacks are like an epidemic. When one girl is possessed, a whole bunch of others end up being possessed'. Another teacher, who had witnessed his fair share of spiritual attacks, speculated that a girl's wails acted 'as a catalyst', setting off the other students. Addressing the crisis generally meant quarantining the possessed girls before their symptoms spread to the rest of the students. According to a science teacher, 'Some girls scream when they are possessed while others start shivering. When I see a student shivering, I isolate her. I know I cannot leave her with the others, or she will contaminate the entire class'. In Dogondoutchi, the 'epidemic' of spirit attacks reportedly has some parents concerned enough that they choose not to send their daughters to schools perceived to be 'infested' with spirits. School principals have mentioned to Masquelier that following a spiritual attack, it is not uncommon for parents to move their daughters (and sometimes even their sons) to other schools to avoid the dreaded possibility they might be targeted by spirits.

Spirit attacks come in waves, and they are unpredictable. A middle school teacher told Masquelier the establishment where he taught natural science was large enough that he would be lecturing in his classroom unaware that in another section of the school, a dozen girls jumped over furniture or fell to the floor, twisting in odd, unnatural ways. During certain periods of the year (especially the hot season that ran from March to May), 'not a week went by without a commotion provoked by stricken girls'. Witnesses to spirit attacks often stress the incredible speed with which the affliction spreads from one girl to the next. 'I was reading out loud the catastrophic grades my students received on a French exam, when girls in the classroom started screaming. I don't know what prompted it. What I know is that when it happens, it comes suddenly then it stops just as suddenly', explained a middle school teacher. 'One girl screams out of the blue. By the time you've reached the door to seek help, three others start acting weird and before you know it, it has spread to half the class', a school principal volunteered. As a form of contagious affliction, 'mass hysteria' highlights the interconnectedness of persons, the centrality of intersubjectivity, and the role of empathy (or emotional resonance). It further suggests that the relevant unit of analysis is not an individual with a problem but

'These Spirit Attacks Are Like an Epidemic'

rather the emergent, contingent, and often ephemeral constellation of people brought together by affective flows and sensed intensities.

Friendship, Permeability and Contagion

Often exposure to a possessed person appears to be a sufficient condition for triggering possession. Emotional closeness likely has a role to play as well. Victims of a spiritual attack are frequently said to be friends. People identify girls who are caught by spirits as the 'popular girls' in school, who gang up against other students or are part of a clique. 'It's usually the same girls who are possessed. They are part of a network. It's like they understand each other', is how a school principal put it. 'When a girl falls, I can tell you who else will be possessed next – those girls who like to show off', a teacher said. In sum, the afflicted appear to share an affective connection. They talk about school, tensions at home, boys; they share tastes, values, styles and opinions on other people (Winkler-Reid 2016). Friends know everything about each other; they 'share everything. This one will be able to tell you stuff [no one else knows] about her friend who was attacked', one former student explained.

In past decades more girls than ever are attending school. As elsewhere in the world where female sociality is largely restricted to the domestic space, schooling has enabled girls to make new connections and strike new friendships, beyond the boundaries of the family or the neighbourhood (Dyson 2010). Making sense of the girls' experience of spirit possession calls for a reconsideration of the place of empathy and intersubjectivity in hysteria outbreaks. Such a move complicates the notions of individual boundedness upon which psychiatric definitions of hysteria are based. An important dimension of friendship is mimetic, Winkler-Reid (2016) posits in her study of girls' friendship in a London school, meaning that friends shape each other according to gendered criteria. Persons are produced out of their social and emotional entanglements with others, studies of friendship demonstrate (Evans 2010; Winkler-Reid 2016). The intersubjective nature of processes of friendship in turn suggests how heightened connectedness between schoolgirls may provide a substrate for possession to spread.

In Niger adolescent girls and young women are widely acknowledged to be fragile, vulnerable, and easily distracted from their religious duties. As such, they are particularly susceptible to intrusive spirits looking to regain some footing in the landscape they previously controlled. 'It's girls who walk around at night who get caught by spirits', a young man told Masquelier, echoing other comments that equate moral laxity with vulnerability to spiritual intrusion. Spirits are said to be attracted to girls who wear close-fitting, skimpy outfits. '*Aljanu* choose girls who expose their bodies. They like beautiful girls', a maths teacher said. The absence of head coverings provides another leitmotif in people's explanations of what makes girls defenceless against spirits. 'When it's hot, the girls don't cover their heads. Or they don't wear hijabs. They leave their hair exposed. That's what attracts the spirits', is how a university student put it. As noted earlier, such explanations are embedded in a larger moral discourse that equates female immodesty with immorality and decadence. In such contexts, the hijab is a signifier of modesty while also constituting a physical shield against spiritual aggression. The protection it exerts is at once symbolic and 'solid', thereby fully discouraging potential spiritual assailants.

Regardless of whether spirits are unwelcome intruders or desired guests, possession in Niger is best understood through the semantics of penetrability and susceptibility.[11] Spirits penetrate human bodies, female bodies in particular, because the latter are inherently porous. Here, the language of permeability indexes at once bodily porousness and moral frailty. Girls and young women are impressionable and easily corruptible. In other words, they are susceptible to what goes on around them, which is why they get 'caught' by *aljanu* just as they might catch measles or meningitis. Understanding possession through the lens of contagion means focusing on affliction as a relational rather than personal phenomenon (Seale-Feldman 2019). As we shall see, since interpretations of spirit attacks are often steeped in a moralizing rhetoric aimed at cultivating feminine virtue, making sense of this pattern of susceptibility to spiritual intrusion requires that we take seriously the Muslim discourse of moral contagion and the spirit-centred narratives of loss, revenge or seduction that are part of a tangle of affective connections surging and swelling and setting things in motion – or simply receding even as they continue to resonate.

'These Spirit Attacks Are Like an Epidemic'

Possession as Imitative Contagion

We owe much of the theorizing on 'social contagion' to Gabriel Tarde, a French social theorist and contemporary of Emile Durkheim, whose work proved instrumental to the development of sociology, psychology and criminology. Contrary to Durkheim who privileged society as a kind of superorganism superseding the individual, Tarde argued that society was made up of individuals (the so-called 'monads') constantly interacting with one another. Tarde's aim was to build a model of society that would account for how 'the many can act as one' while still preserving diversity and difference. Rejecting both individual psychology and social determinism, Tarde described the self as a 'socialized monad' (Candea 2010: 12) that was open to the influence of external factors while society was 'a tissue of inter-spiritual actions' (Tarde 2018: 11). In this model of society, people were not understood to be isolated units but nodes of intersection between diverse lines of imitation (Barry and Thrift 2007; Tarde 1969). Tarde was interested in the lines of imitation (or communication) that connected subjects rather than the subjects themselves (Blackman 2007).

Tarde noticed how remarkably open (or susceptible) to one another people were. They appeared to embrace, almost in the manner of hypnotic suggestion, the ideas, beliefs and practices of others, and later discarded, replicated or modified them accordingly. Beliefs, desires and behaviours thus spread (at times quickly) across populations as if they were infectious, yet they also interacted with one another just as ripples in a pond would if two stones were dropped in different places (King 2016). Eschewing the notion of pre-existing social structures, Tarde identified imitation as the basic modality of social action. More than simple mimicry, imitation referred to people's receptivity to the influence of the surrounding social world. A new idea could spread across populations and 'crystallize' so that it became habit or custom while others failed to stick even as they affected people. By privileging imitation and interaction, Tarde put the accent on the contingent, fluid and undetermined nature of social processes. To quote Bruno Latour and Vincent Lépinay (2009: 42), in Tarde's epidemiological model of society, 'all is imitation, multiplicity and repetition but the latter are guided by no plan, no dialectic, no finality'.

Tarde's work provides a useful starting point for considering the role of exposure (or contagion) in the spread of social phenomena such as mass possession. His theory of imitation, in particular, can help us articulate the collective experience of trance in Nigerien schools as relational phenomena in their own right rather than the individualized expression of deep-seated conflicts. In a well-known passage (cited in the epigraph), Tarde asserts that imitation is strikingly similar to somnambulism, a mode of partial awareness fuelled by collective waves of affect in which the focus is on the power of suggestion. By putting forward a compliant subject, where no '"real" self exists prior to mimesis' (Leys in Blackman 2007: 585), the mimetic model elucidates the ways that schoolgirls can affect and be affected by each other so powerfully.[12] Such a model accounts for the spontaneous nature of spiritual attacks and their temporal clustering (occurring as in waves, a pattern people often comment on), while accommodating the diverse personal histories of the victims.

If, for Tarde, society instantiates a generalized condition of mimetic resonance, the crowd turns out to be the 'perfect and absolute' (1962: 70) form of sociality: the minute one person comes up with an idea, it will be transmitted immediately to everyone else, bypassing reason and criticality. Like the crowd, a classroom of possessed girls (whose members mimic and amplify each other's impulses and actions) operates according to the logic of suggestibility: the screams of one girl will trigger mimetic behaviour in the others. The influence the girls exert on one another is so forceful, magnetic, that they can be said to entrance each other. The only difference between mass possession and ordinary forms of contagion (such as in friendship) is the intensity of suggestibility the subjects are under. To explain this further, let us turn to the spirits themselves.

Haunted Schools

Before being assimilated to the jinn of the Qur'an, local spirits were known in Hausa as *iskoki* (singular *iska*). Since spirits were both the source of and the remedy for human suffering, no human project could succeed without their support. Akin to the wind (*iska*), after which they were named, *iskoki* were mysterious, powerful and occasionally fearful creatures, but they were not perceived as straightforwardly evil, though they could be vindictive, even cruel. They routinely intervened in human affairs to upset the course of events or to restore order where there was once havoc. The advent of drought, a wave of sickness, ruined crops or vulnerability to an impending enemy attack were often attributed to them: the *iskoki* felt slighted and were avenging themselves by causing human suffering. Appeasing them and securing their support required providing them with the sacrificial blood upon which they fed. While today fewer people make routine offerings to the *iskoki* to guarantee health, security and prosperity, many nevertheless remain wary of the harm neglected spirits may visit on communities, households or individuals.

Spiritual retaliation is the language people frequently draw on to account for the surges of sickness plaguing large numbers of adolescent schoolgirls. The jinn are said to be angry for having been mistreated. During spiritual attacks (and occasionally exorcisms), as they 'borrow' the voice of their unwitting hosts, they often mention having lost their homes when new schools or classrooms were built. Narratives centring on cut trees and lost abodes are so widespread that few question their veracity. As they circulate among households and neighbourhoods, they are 'possessed by the memories of other people's experiences' (Steedly 1993: 22) and become recognizable, real – strange yet sensible. To quote Mary Steedly (1993: 23), these narratives are 'as much "about" other stories as they are about events, real or imagined'. A former student recounted what happened at the middle school he once attended in Dogondoutchi:

> One year the spirits possessed four girls. One of them, Salamatou, could not study ever again. The girls were possessed by spirits who used to live in the place before the *collège* [middle school] was built in 1977. People cut the tree where the spirits resided. Now [the spirits] possess girls intermittently. It happened in 2006, in 2008, and in 2010. The 7th and 8th grade classrooms. Only the girls.

Across wide swaths of land, the aggressive clearing of the bush that accompanied urban expansion, the shift towards individual property, and the spread of Islam translated into the dislocation of indigenous spirits. Trees, which anchored spirits to particular places, were cut down to make way for roads, farms and human settlements

(Luxereau and Roussel 1997). Having lost their anchorage yet unwilling to leave, these spirits now sulkily hover over the places they once called home. Increasingly they manifest themselves by taking possession of adolescent schoolgirls. In the former student's testimony, the simple reference to the felled trees (to make space for classrooms) conjures a vision of the *collège* as a space saturated with sorrow and rage, an affective vortex whose pulsing intensities drew in unsuspecting girls and often locked them in, ultimately short-circuiting their dreams of social mobility.

At a fundamental level, the mass possession on school grounds recapitulates a complex history of loss, neglect and disaffection. While the erasure of the spiritscape often coincides in the moral imagination with the experience of colonization in the first half of the last century, it is more accurate to trace such transformations to the post-independence period during which people massively converted to Islam (Masquelier 2001).[13] In Arewa, the Hausa-speaking district where Masquelier has been conducting fieldwork since 1988, people allegedly started 'forgetting' the spirits when they officially adopted Islam practices. Muslim identity became synonymous with status, social mobility and respectability, while *l'animisme* (French-speaking Nigeriens use the term to describe spirit veneration) was increasingly associated with backwardness, rusticity and ignorance. Embracing ways of being Muslim (praying, fasting, giving their children Muslim names and so on) gave people access to social and material resources non-Muslims were largely denied.

Seeking to purify Islam from *animisme*, *malamai* (Muslim religious specialists, scholars, teachers) destroyed altars, demonized guardian spirits and forbid the enactment of communal rituals aimed at securing spiritual support. In Arewa, Muslim factions put a stop to the performance of ceremonies designed to purge (or protect) towns and villages from pestilence. In the late 1980s, some residents of Dogondoutchi lamented that the loss of traditions, particularly the abandonment of *gyaran gari*, a ritual aimed at enlisting the tutelary spirits' protection against sickness, resulted in a resurgence of seasonal epidemics.[14] The promotion of Muslim ways of being and the language of purification used by Muslim preachers working to eradicate spirit veneration facilitated land appropriation. Trees were no longer part of the wider cosmological fabric. They

'These Spirit Attacks Are Like an Epidemic'

were just 'things'. In Dogondoutchi, a Sufi preacher gained fame for chasing a spirit from her abode – she was said to reside in a tree on a land parcel everyone avoided – so he could build a mosque as part of his efforts to revivify the faith (Masquelier 2009).

With the spread of Izala, facilitated by the state's retreat from social services in structurally adjusted Niger, the proliferation of accessible media technologies and the sense of 'abjection' (Ferguson 1999: 236) experienced by young marginalized men who felt cheated out of post-independence promises of prosperity, Islamic iconoclasm intensified. Amidst worrisome unemployment, rising social inequalities and accelerated rural exodus, Izala gave voice to a host of moral concerns while offering disenfranchised populations a framework for collective action. Importantly, it provided an Islamic alternative to secular models of nationhood, family and sociality, actively shaping the emerging Nigerien public sphere in the process. Questions of Muslim identity (and religiosity) acquired a new salience while spirit-centred practices were forcibly denounced.[15]

Izala leaders urged people to ignore signs and symptoms of spiritual intervention and concentrate on the performance of daily prayers. Under no circumstances, they warned, should recourse for serious afflictions be sought from exorcists or 'animists'. Sickness was within the strict purview of biomedicine. Since spirits play a central role in social reproduction, women who sought their protection – or sought protection from them – to ensure successful pregnancies, shield themselves from jealous co-wives and preserve the stability of their marriage were particularly affected by the reformist Muslim ban on spirit-based therapies.

Given how often people mention forgotten spirits, destroyed altars and abandoned rituals, it would be reasonable to assume that *aljanu* are simply gone. As many will tell you, however, the spirits have not disappeared. One might even argue that by demonizing *aljanu*, Islamic iconoclasm paradoxically created the conditions for their reappearance. By equating spirits with evil, reformist Muslim preachers ultimately attributed powers to them, including the power to corrupt. Far from becoming irrelevant, *aljanu* today remain vital to the definition of Islam, even if, for some, they are forever outside its grasp. What is more, they routinely remind people of their presence. Some roam the roads that unfurl across the landscape, provoking accidents and prompting travellers to avoid certain spots

(Masquelier 2002). In Zinder, Niger's second largest town, an *aljana* (female spirit) displaced by sprawling human settlements was once rumoured to wander the streets in search of men she could proposition (Masquelier 2008). In other cities, *génies tchatcheurs* allegedly rove about in hordes, ravaging girls and terrorizing neighbourhoods. And throughout Niger, secondary schools have become the haunting grounds of bitter, revengeful spirits claiming they lived there long before people arrived. 'The spirits' attacks started ever since they built our school', a high school teacher told Masquelier. 'Now we are used to it.'

Today the presence of spirits is almost always understood through the lens of the past – a past that puts constraints on the present. 'The school where I teach has been haunted for many years', a maths teacher confessed. 'We make sure the students avoid certain places on the school grounds. We don't want them to get hurt' (latrines must be avoided for spirits are known to congregate in 'dirty' places). Parents and former students we spoke with evoked a past infiltrating the present in the form of a menace looming over schools such that before possession attacks even took place, they were already anticipated as the inevitable offshoots – the never-ending ripples – of a violent, iconoclastic past.

At one level the violence of the past leaves tangible traces. It contaminates schools, turning them into 'toxic' places that must be periodically cleansed by religious specialists. At another level, as we shall see, it produces what we refer to as 'affective contagion', a web of intersubjective influence and susceptibility. In Tardean fashion, ideas, stories, emotions about spirits, their biographies and the revengeful actions spread wave-like across society through processes of replication and difference. Although these waves have their origins in individual events, they also gain their own momentum and force (Sampson 2012), a force which can be dissipated or amplified, and can even merge with other waves to create the intense climate of effervescence that translates into mass possession.

The Promises and Perils of Schooling

In Niger, the least literate country on the planet, girls' education is routinely advertised by the government, rights associations and private citizens as a critical dimension of national development. 'When a girl goes to school, the whole country matures', goes a well-known aphorism taught to schoolchildren. By implying a correspondence between the national body and the bodies of schoolgirls, the aphorism is a reminder that girls' education often serves as the gage for assessing Niger's position along a scale of unilinear progress. This model of development presumes that education constitutes a guaranteed path to social mobility. By the same token, when girls forego schooling to marry, they are robbed of their aspirations, agency and economic capital (World Bank 2018). Schools are imagined as the systematic solution to many of the problems that currently plague Niger (high rates of early marriage, a galloping demography, a low literacy rate, stark gender inequalities, poverty and so on). Niger, which leads the world in early marriage and population growth, has been the target of multiple externally funded initiatives designed to promote girls' (especially teenage girls') education. By lengthening the interval between the onset of puberty and the advent of marriage, these initiatives focus on rescuing girlhood from 'oppressive' patriarchal norms and give girls time to develop before they assume the cloak of adulthood. Yet, by presuming that schooling inevitably produces agentive individuals who, through the right mix of hard work and commitment, fulfil their aspirations of social mobility, this model of development (which international lenders, such as the World Bank, aggressively promote) often obscures the multiple challenges adolescent female students living in a poor country like Niger face in school.

Teenage girls' education in Niger is mired in controversy. Though education is now mandatory between the ages of seven and fifteen, many girls are pulled out of school before their fifteenth birthday. Among those who remain in school, relatively few ultimately complete their education. Amid widespread talk, fuelled by national and international NGOs, that education is a 'human right' which no girl should be deprived of, a coalition of Muslim religious associations has publicly denounced adolescent girls' secular education, advocating marriage as the proper alternative. When a bill aimed at protecting the rights of girls to attend school up to eighteen was submitted to the National Assembly in 2012, its members overwhelmingly rejected it. Islamic association leaders had labelled the bill 'satanic' and 'contrary to Islamic teachings'. The National Assembly's *députés* feared what would happen should they approve such a bill, given the political clout these religious leaders enjoyed.

At the heart of the controversy lies the issue of sexual promiscuity, which opponents of adolescent girls' education argue is fostered by the schools' inadequate curriculum, secularist agenda and failure to segregate students by gender. While many parents believe that a high school degree may lead to a prosperous future[16] and daughters with stable incomes typically provide generously for their aging parents,[17] they also fret about the dangers adolescent girls face in school, given the prevalence of sexual harassment and sexual improprieties. Moreover, in the eyes of some parents, Western secular education is not conducive to the development of the proper Muslim wife, respectful, compliant, and devoted to her husband. Added to the fact that mothers whose daughters attend school cannot rely on their labour, parents fear that knowledge will make girls 'bossy', proud, and unwilling to perform their duties. Village parents also worry about sending adolescent girls away to school given the risks they confront while living in town with little or no supervision. Schools are sometimes criticized for giving girls too much licence. Occurring in contexts saturated by what Michel de Certeau (2005) calls *langage de l'inquiétude* (language of apprehension), the frequent outbreaks of collective trance in schools fuel parental concerns about the suitability of schooling for post-pubescent girls.

Affective Contagion

As Aidan Seale-Feldman (2019: 321) observed, the so-called phenomenon of mass hysteria 'confounds assumptions of what an affliction is', for rather than being bounded within one individual, 'it moves and travels, and appears and disappears'. Drawing on Tarde's work on social contagion, we have suggested that a focus on relationality and suggestibility offers a useful analytics for considering how mass hysteria precisely operates. The stories, confessions, memories, feelings, knowledges and practices having to do with womanhood, schooling and spirits that circulate across the social landscape have widespread, yet also intimate effects on people's lives, especially schoolgirls. Tracing these effects amidst the tangle of 'exchanges, misunderstandings, and manipulations'

(Mayneri 2018: 883) that characterizes secular and religious discourse in Niger is challenging, for these effects are 'rooted not in fixed conditions of possibility but in the actual lines of potential that a *something* coming together calls to mind and sets in motion' (Stewart 2007: 2). Which of these feed the circuits of transmission or, conversely, stall, disperse only to get picked up again and surge? Kathleen Stewart's concept of 'ordinary affects' comes closest to capturing these surging capacities that work 'not through "meaning" per se, but rather through the way they pick up density and texture as they move through bodies, dreams, dramas, and social worldings of all kinds' (Stewart 2007: 3).

Stewart defines ordinary affects as feelings that circulate publicly but also powerfully infiltrate intimate lives. Ordinary affects, she argues, are 'more directly compelling than ideologies, as well as more fractious, multiplicitous, and unpredictable than symbolic meanings' (2007: 3). Rather than lending themselves to clear-cut definition and classification, ordinary affects are diffuse, emergent, flighty, inconsistent – 'a tangle of potential connections' (2007: 4). They are at once abstract and concrete, immanent yet also inconsistent. Because they exist in a state of potentiality and resonance, they cannot be neatly captured in a single plane of analysis and must instead by mapped through distinct, yet synchronized registers and representations.

Take, for instance, the discourse of dissipation and impiety many Muslim preachers draw on to account for mass possession in schools. With their bare heads and revealing garments, adolescent girls constitute a temptation for lecherous spirits, these preachers have argued in their sermons, as they enjoin girls and women to veil. By claiming that women's immodesty heightens their susceptibility to spiritual attacks and the hijab is the most effective protection against such attacks, they construct female subjects, especially unmarried girls, simultaneously as objects of anxiety and vehicles of redemption. These diagnoses and recommendations in turn aggregate, intersect, resonate or conflict with other images, stories, conversations and experiences centred on spirits, schoolgirls, haunted schools and hijabs to constitute an animate circuit or what Raymond Williams called structures of feeling. The latter need not be articulated or rationalized to 'exert palpable pressures' (Williams 1977: 132). One might describe it as an instance of affective contagion.

How this tangle of pathways and disjunctures snaps into sense or resonates with other scenes, images and experiences in some ill-defined ways is difficult to trace. For instance, how does the anticipation of failing an exam intersect with the more insidious sense that the classroom is haunted? The lines of resonances and connection crystallize most sharply when they produce, in a paroxysm of grief and energy, the loud and not always coherent recriminations of spirits who blame people for their homelessness, point the finger at sexily dressed girls they fell attracted to, insult school supervisors, or threaten to kill teachers and students. That they remain blurred, unsteady is a reminder that as Janice Boddy (1989: 15) observed, 'possession has numerous significances and countless implications'. We must be cautious not to overdetermine intent or outcome. By relying on the language of contagion, we have sought to apprehend the relational dimension of mass possession without closing off paths of questioning or sources of ambiguity that contribute to the affective linkages and vibrating intensities coursing through (and resonating across) bodies, schoolyards and neighbourhoods.

Concluding Thoughts

Observers often use the concept of contagion metaphorically to invoke processes of cultural diffusion or point to the social configuration of noncommunicable diseases. When Nigeriens speak of spirit possession spreading among schoolgirls *like an epidemic*, they are speaking literally. The following testimony drives the point further home. A friend once recounted how, during a spiritual attack in a schoolyard in 2010, several girls started screaming and foaming at the mouth. Everyone scampered to escape the wrathful jinn, except for one teacher. She bravely stood up to one of the possessing jinn, who said she was grieving the loss of her husband, killed during the construction of a school wall. '[The teacher] was immune to the spirit's action', is how our friend put it. The teacher had inherited an *aljani* who shielded her from the nefarious impact of jinn lurking on school grounds, under large trees or on the edge of the bush. 'Had she not been protected by her *aljani na gida*, the spirit would have most probably killed her', our friend concluded. Immunity was the concept our friend drew on to describe the teacher's imperviousness to the threat posed by the revengeful spirit. In the way it gestures to not only empathy and permeability but also immunity and resistance, the language of contagion is well suited to capture the contingent, unstable, yet impactful patterns of affective communicability that psychiatrists refer to as 'mass hysteria'.

By examining the phenomenon of spirit possession through the analytical lens of contagion, we have sought to capture something of the ways in which Nigerien schoolgirls are affected by one another and by the wider social landscape in which they navigate. The analytics of contagion shift the focus from possessed subjects (as self-contained entities) to the interconnectedness of selves by pointing to processes of emotional resonance, 'interaffectivity' (Fuch 2017), mutuality and attunement. In other words, it puts the accent on the mimetic, relational dimensions of personhood, manifesting 'continuity with other persons' while disregarding the forensic individuality, manifesting 'temporal continuity in the life of the person' (Lambek 2013: 849), on which psychiatry is based. Eschewing models of subjectivism and somatization and framing our discussion of trance around concepts of interaction, exposure and haunting has enabled us to align it more closely with Nigeriens' understanding of mass possession.

Drawing on the work of Tarde, who theorized how social actors exert deep power over one another through diverse interactive and imitative processes, we tentatively sketched some of the webs of connectedness in which schoolgirls can be said to function as 'monadic singularities'. Exploring the relational aspects of spirit possession, we argued, implies a consideration of how discourses on spiritual attacks, girls' education and morality are entangled in a prediscursive flow of contagious affects and energies. Such flows of ideas, feelings and narratives exist in circuits of connectivity and ruptures, contributing to the emergence of a mood that is 'neither precisely of self nor of the world' (Throop 2014). As instances of what Stewart called 'ordinary affects', they help shape ritual engagement, ethical orientations as well as ordinary embodied practices in diffuse, impersonal yet effective ways. By tracing some of the ideas, narratives, emotions and images that circulate along multiple pathways, gain momentum to later amplify or dissipate, we have attempted to shed light on the contagious landscape of possession in Niger, pointing to the tangle of potential linkages and zones of contact between spiritual forces and permeable bodies, religious heritage, educational models, hijabs and hauntings.

Acknowledgements

The long-term research grounding this chapter was undertaken by Adeline Masquelier and funded by grants from Tulane University, the National Science Foundation, the Wenner-Gren Foundation, the National Institute of Mental Health and the National Geographic Society. When Masquelier met Abouzeidi Maidouka and Ly Belko, both were completing an MA in gender and development. Maidouka was writing a thesis on spirit possession. This chapter is the fruit of a collaboration that began in 2018. We are deeply indebted to the people in Niger who participated in this research. We thank the editors, Lotte Meinert and Jens Seeberg, and the external reviewers for their helpful editorial suggestions.

Adeline Masquelier
Professor, Department of Anthropology
Tulane University, US

Abouzeidi Maidouka Dillé
Consultant
Niger

Ly Amadou H. Belko
Consultant
Niger

Notes

1. During possession, each human host is possessed by a distinct spirit. Spirits come and go, however. Hence, the same spirit can possess several people consecutively. Spirits known as *génies tchatcheurs* are said to operate in bands, though reports sometimes mention a single spirit causing mischief.
2. In the two cases we know of that involved boys, the spirits were *na gida*, 'family spirits' inherited from deceased kin. Such spirits cannot be exorcized. Instead, a sacrifice must be made to placate them. Victims may choose to undergo initiation to formalize their lifelong commitment to these spirits.

3. An instructor admitted he occasionally continued lecturing while the possessed girls were rolling and writhing on the floor. These crises happened so often he saw no point in cancelling classes.
4. A science teacher estimated that during the hot season there were approximately three to four 'incidents' a week in the school where he taught, though few resulted in the entire school shutting down.
5. Being bereft of substance, spirits take control of fleshly bodies to materialize themselves – that is, to acquire physicality and, importantly, a voice with which to utter grievances, convey desires, command and warn.
6. Izala, which is short for Jama'atu Izalat al-Bid'a wa Iqamat al-Sunna (Society for the Removal of Innovation and the Restoration of Tradition), originated in Nigeria out of dissatisfaction with local Muslims' alleged ignorance of Islam (Loimeier 1997).
7. Due partly to press coverage, *génies tchatcheurs* enjoyed a great deal of attention early on. Today they are often assimilated in the national imagination with the evicted spirits seeking reparations on school grounds. Though both categories of spirits possess schoolgirls, they are driven by different motives and have distinct modus operandi.
8. Whether or not they are manufactured abroad, tightly fitted, revealing clothes are assumed to be inspired by Western fashions. As such, they embody the very values (secularism, immodesty, conspicuous consumption and so on) Izala and other Muslim organizations have been actively campaigning against.
9. Healthcare in Niger suffers from an insufficiently developed infrastructure, a chronic lack of resources and a dismally low number of medical practitioners relative to population.
10. Some of them travel great distances to avail themselves of the services of proficient exorcists. Others opt for 'digital' exorcism, taking advantage of the emergence of a new crop of ritual experts claiming they can expel spirits at a distance through the use of cell phones.
11. During ceremonies held to promote individual and communal well-being, the sharp clatter of calabash drums, the wails of the monochord violin and the songs of praise singers attract spirits, inviting them to possess human hosts (Masquelier 2001).
12. Social contagion is thus incompatible with the idea of the self-contained, rational calculating actor.
13. Niger gained its independence in 1960.
14. Performed during the cold season, *gyaran gari* insulated communities from the threat of communicable diseases, such as measles and meningitis, brought from the outside.
15. To foster a return to 'authentic' Islam, Izala leaders also denounced practices that had long been part of Muslim people's life, such as the veneration of saintly Muslim figures, the recitation of Sufi prayer formulas and the use of Qur'anic *materia medica*.

16. The economic downturn of the past decades, associated with high rates of unemployment among educated youth, has tarnished the image of schooling as the guaranteed ticket to high-paying jobs.
17. Daughters are widely believed to take better care of their parents than sons, regardless of their respective financial circumstances.

References

Barry, Andrew, and Nigel Thrift. 2007. 'Gabriel Tarde: Imitation, Invention, and Economy', *Economy and Society* 36(4): 509–25.
Blackman, Lisa. 2007. 'Reinventing Psychological Matters: The Importance of the Suggestive Realm in Tarde's Ontology', *Economy and Society* 36(4): 574–96.
Boddy, Janice. 1989. *Wombs and Alien Spirits: Women, Men, and the Zar Cult in Northern Sudan*. Madison: University of Wisconsin Press.
Candea, Matei (ed.). 2010. *The Social after Gabriel Tarde*. London: Routledge.
Certeau, Michel de. 2005. *La Possession de Loudun*. Paris: Gallimard-Julliard.
Dyson, Jane. 2010. 'Friendship in Practice: Girls' Work in the Indian Himalayas', *American Ethnologist* 37: 482–98.
Espírito Santo, Diana, and Ruy Blanes. 2014. 'Introduction', in Ruy Blanes and Diana Espírito Santo (eds), *The Social Life of Spirits*. Chicago: Chicago University Press, pp. 1–32.
Evans, Gillian. 2010. 'The Value of Friendship: Subject/Object Transformations in the Economy of Becoming a Person (Bermondsey, Southeast London)', in Amit Desai and Evan Killick (eds), *The Ways of Friendship: Anthropological Perspectives*. Oxford: Berghahn Books, pp. 174–96.
Ferguson, James. 1999. *Expectations of Modernity: Myths and Meanings of Urban Life on the Zambian Copperbelt*. Berkeley: University of California Press.
Fuch, Thomas. 2017. 'Intercorporeality and Interaffectivity', in Christian Meyer, Jürgen Streeck and J. Scott Jordan (eds), *Intercorporeality: Emerging Socialities in Interaction*. New York: Oxford University Press, pp. 194–209.
Hodgson, Dorothy. 1997. 'Embodying the Contradictions of Modernity: Gender and Spirit Possession among Maasai in Tanzania', in Maria Grosz-Ngate and Omari H. Kokole (eds), *Gendered Encounters: Challenging Cultural Boundaries and Social Hierarchies in Africa*. New York: Routledge, pp. 111–29.
King, Anthony. 2016. 'Gabriel Tarde and Contemporary Social Theory', *Sociological Theory* 34(1): 45–61.
Lambek, Michael. 2013. 'The Continuous and Discontinuous Person: Two Dimensions of Ethical Life', *Journal of the Royal Anthropological Institute* 19(4): 837–58.

Latour, Bruno, and Vincent Antonin Lépinay. 2009. *The Science of Passionate Interest: An Introduction to Gabriele Tarde's Economic Anthropology*. Chicago: Prickly Paradigm Press.

Loimeier, Roman. 1997. *Islamic Reform and Political Change in Northern Nigeria*. Evanston, IL: Northwestern University Press.

Luxereau, Anne, and Bernard Roussel. 1997. *Changements Écologiques et Sociaux au Niger: Des Interactions Étroites*. Paris: L'Harmattan.

Mahmood, Saba. 2005. *Politics of Piety: The Islamic Revival and the Feminist Subject*. Princeton, NJ: Princeton University Press.

Masquelier, Adeline. 2001. *Prayer Has Spoiled Everything: Possession, Power, and Identity in an Islamic Town of Niger*. Durham, NC: Duke University Press.

―――. 2002. 'Road Mythographies: Space, Mobility, and the Historical Imagination in Postcolonial Niger', *American Ethnologist* 29(4): 829–56.

―――. 2008. 'When Female Spirits Start Veiling: The Case of the Veiled She-Devil in a Muslim Town of Niger', *Africa Today* 54(3): 38–64.

―――. 2009. *Women and Islamic Revival in a West African Town*. Bloomington: Indiana University Press.

―――. 2018. 'Schooling, Spirit Possession, and the "Modern Girl" in Niger', in Muriel Gomez-Perez (ed.), *Femmes d'Afrique et Émancipations: Entre Normes Sociales Contraignantes et Nouveaux Possibles*. Paris: Karthala, pp. 299–323.

―――. 2020. 'A Matter of Time: Spirit Possession and the Temporalities of School in Niger', *Journal of Africana Religions* 7(1): 243–66.

Mayneri, Andrea Ceriana. 2018. 'Les Impasses de la Transe à l'École: Violences de Genre, Religions et Protestations à N'Djamena', *Cahiers d'Études Africaines* LVIII (3–4): 881–911.

Meinert, Lotte, and Susan Reynolds Whyte. 2017. '"These Things Continue": Violence as Contamination in Everyday Life after War in Northern Uganda', *Ethos* 45(2): 271–86.

Niandou-Souley, Abdoulaye, and Gado Alzouma. 1996. 'Islamic Renewal in Niger: From Monolith to Plurality', *Social Compass* 43(2): 240–65.

O'Brien, Susan. 2001. 'Spirit Discipline: Gender, Islam, and Hierarchies of Treatment in Post-Colonial Northern Nigeria', *Interventions: The International Journal of Post-Colonial Studies* 3: 222–24.

Ong, Aihwa. 1988. 'The Production of Possession: Spirits and the Multinational Corporation in Malaysia', *American Ethnologist* 15(1): 28–42.

Oumar, Issoufou Adamou. 2019. 'Santé/Troubles de Conversion ou Hystérie de Conversion: Les Explications Scientifiques sur le Phénomène du "Génie Tchatcheur" et ses Conséquences', *Le Sahel*, 5 September, 9. Retrieved 15 January 2020 from http//www.lesahel.org/.

Sampson, Tony D. 2012. *Virality*. Minneapolis: University of Minnesota Press.

Seale-Feldman, Aidan. 2019. 'Relational Affliction: Reconceptualizing "Mass Hysteria"', *Ethos* 47(3): 307–25.

Sharp, Lesley. 1990. 'Possessed and Dispossessed Youth: Spirit Possession of School Children in Northwest Madagascar', *Culture, Medicine, and Psychiatry* 14: 339–64.

———. 1993. *The Possessed and the Dispossessed: Spirits, Identity, and Power in a Madagascar Migrant Town*. Berkeley: University of California Press.

Smith, James H. 2001. 'Of Spirit Possession and Structural Adjustment Programs: Government Downsizing, Education and their Enchantments in Neo-Liberal Kenya', *Journal of Religion in Africa* 31(4): 427–56.

Steedly, Mary Margaret. 1993. *Hanging without a Rope: Narrative Experience in Colonial and Postcolonial Karoland*. Princeton, NJ: Princeton University Press.

Stewart, Kathleen. 2007. *Ordinary Affects*. Durham, NC: Duke University Press.

Tarde, Gabriel de. 1962. *The Laws of Imitation*, trans. Elsie Clews Parsons. Gloucester, MA: Peter Smith.

———. 1969. *On Communication and Social Influence: Selected Papers*, ed. Terry N. Clark. Chicago: University of Chicago Press.

———. 2018. *Psychologie Economique*, vol. I. Paris: Hachette.

Throop, Jason. 2014. 'Moral Moods', *Ethos* 42(1): 65–83.

Williams, Raymond. 1977. *Marxism and Literature*. New York: Oxford University Press.

Winkler-Reid, Sarah. 2016. 'Friendship, Bitching, and the Making of Ethical Selves: What It Means to Be a Good Friend among Girls in a London School', *Journal of the Royal Anthropological Institute* 22(1): 166–82.

World Bank. 2018. *World Bank Education Overview: Girls' Education*. Washington, DC: World Bank Group. Retrieved 19 January 2020 from http://documents.worldbank.org/curated/en/924471541079772899/World-Bank-Education-Overview-Girls-Education.

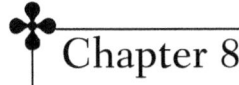
Chapter 8
Haunted by Internet Porn
Configuration of a Hidden Contagion

Douglas Hollan

In the thirty years I have been practising as an anthropologist and as a research psychoanalyst,[1] I have never worked with a person whose primary presenting problem was an addiction to or compulsive involvement with sexually oriented internet sites. However, I have met several men who, although initially complaining about such things as depression, anxiety, or various family and social problems, eventually found a way of telling me about their viewing of internet 'porn' and the impact this viewing has had on their social, emotional and erotic lives.[2] Without exception, these revelations were embarrassing for the men involved. And without exception, all of the men felt contaminated and affected by the images they had been exposed to, in the sense that they could not easily *not* think about them once exposed to them and in the sense that they had great difficulty abstaining from further viewing. While there were significant differences in the kinds of sexual images and activities the men were attracted to, what was similar across cases was their strong ambivalence towards the images: on the one hand, the men found the images intensely attractive and pleasurable, especially when used to stimulate or accompany masturbation, but on the other hand, they were also disturbed by the sense that they were being seduced and manipulated by the images in some way, and by their lack of control over their own responsiveness to those images.

What all of these men had in common, then, and what made them different from many of the other men and women I have worked with as a research psychoanalyst, is a particular susceptibility to an environmental influence, in this case internet porn, with parallels to the way certain populations are more or less susceptible or vulnerable to infectious agents of one kind or another, or to other kinds of environmental and lifestyle influences. This kind of contagion or social influence is complicated, though, because not only are the men selectively responsive to the vast number of sexual and erotic images available on the internet, this reservoir of images is in turn affected by their selective browsing. Website owners and managers respond to selective browsing by 'thickening' the content and variety of the material that is accessed while pruning that which is not, a dynamic and interactive process that is reminiscent of the way neural connections are thickened and pruned in response to social experience, and one in which no part of the process – neither the men nor the reservoir of images and fantasies – remains stable or unaffected.

I should be clear at the outset that I am using the term 'porn' in its colloquial sense, the sense in which my subjects were using it, to refer to almost any kind of sexually explicit image, not in its dictionary or legal sense. I should also be clear that I am referring here to a very particular subset of people who view porn, those for whom the viewing has become a highly repetitive, obsessive-like activity that leaves them feeling that they have little or no control over such viewing. As I indicate later, porn viewing is widespread among both men and women of all ages, and for most, it is not problematic in the way I am discussing in this chapter: it does not lead to highly repetitive viewing, it does not lead to intrusive thoughts and images, it does not lead to a haunting sense of contamination, and it does not detract from or impede intimate relationships or other valued activities. In other words, porn viewing may be used and assimilated in many different ways and have many different consequences for people, depending on how it is configured within a person's life and circumstances. The ambivalence towards porn that the men whom I discuss feel is not because they are prudish or because they have negative attitudes – moral, religious or otherwise – towards porn or sexuality per se, but because they have come to realize that their obsessive-like viewing of porn has had some negative consequences for them.

In the remainder of this chapter, I argue that these men's interest in and susceptibility to internet porn was configured by three primary factors: (1) a tendency to be aroused and stimulated by erotic and sexually oriented images, a tendency shared by most if not all humans; (2) a social and professional class standing that enabled them to view and access internet porn easily and privately, and without fear of being caught; and (3) a history of family conflict or trauma that profoundly affected the development of their sexual and erotic lives. I use 'configuring' here in the sense proposed by Meinert and Seeberg in their Introduction to this volume, and by Seeberg and Meinert (2015), to identify and then foreground and underscore the *primary* social and environmental dynamics that collaborate and entangle when social contagions or epidemics emerge. As they point out, configuration analysis resembles contextualization in some ways, 'but, whereas a context analysis is potentially endless (Dilley 1999), configuration analysis is an attempt to foreground certain figures and relations and their influence'. I begin by examining the first two elements of the configuration before using case studies of family conflict and trauma to illustrate how the configuration and entanglement of the elements as a whole played out in the lives of two men. Although the overall number of clinical cases that inform this work is limited, and although I have room to discuss only two of these cases in detail, I have every reason to believe that the kind of obsessive internet use and its dysphoric effects I describe here are more widespread than is usually imagined, and that in this respect, it resembles other forms of social and material contagion in which the phenomenon or experience that is spreading or being transmitted is not readily observable from the third person point of view and may be concealed with relative ease.

Attraction to Sexual Images and Fantasies

In *Civilization and Its Discontents*, Freud (2010) argues that humans must learn to repress innate drives and instincts for sex and aggression (among others) in order to live in social groups, and that this repression of desire inevitably results in frustration and unhappiness. Coincidentally, it also results in the development of a sense of conscience, which Freud referred to as the 'superego', from which people may come to feel guilty and ashamed for even thinking or fantasizing about acting on some of their desires. Yet such repression of desire is never completely successful, and Freud also suggests that many fantasies arise as an imaginary form of compensation for the denial and suppression of the drives and instincts per se. In contrast, other psychoanalysts, including Susan Isaacs (1952) and Melanie Klein (1964, 1975), have suggested that fantasies are an essential component of almost any human thought or action, whether they accompany and inform the expression of a drive or its repression or not.[3] Regardless, though, most psychoanalysts would agree that people fantasize about their lives, whether they eventually act on those fantasies or not, and that this includes fantasizing about sex and other kinds of erotic behaviour.

While Freud argued that all people everywhere have strong sexual and aggressive instincts and that all people everywhere have sexual and aggressive fantasies, Gananath Obeyesekere has raised the question of what role cultures, technologies and institutions play in articulating, suppressing, exploiting or denying human fantasies and imaginative thoughts, including sexually oriented ones. In *Medusa's Hair* (1981), Obeyesekere accepts Freud's view that humans must inevitably learn to suppress and repress themselves in order to live in social groups, and that it is this denial of action and impulse that gives rise to fantasy. He then contrasts the fate of fantasy in places like Sri Lanka and 'the West'. In Sri Lanka, he argues, fantasy is nurtured and given free rein through traditional idioms of iconography, ritual and religious belief. Impulse and action are certainly denied in various ways, but fantasy is allowed and even encouraged to flourish. In the West, however, where harsh work, achievement and 'performance' principles often prevail, fantasy is curtailed and denigrated almost as much as certain impulses and actions per se. As a result, the fantasy that does arise tends to be idiosyncratic, infantile or even perverse.

Obeyesekere's point that the ways in which fantasy becomes stimulated or suppressed, and the meanings and consequences of this for other forms of social and cultural life, have been woefully understudied is well taken (see also Gammeltoft 2014). But I think many internet marketers, researchers and viewers would disagree with his contention that fantasy does not find cultural outlet and elaboration in places like the United States (cf. Caughey 1984; Lindholm 2001: 177), as that is of course exactly what many media and internet products, outlets and websites explicitly cater to. And they would certainly not need Freud to tell them that many people are attracted to sexual images and fantasies, since sexually oriented websites have proliferated since the inception of the internet. While it remains unclear exactly what percentage of the internet and its usage are devoted to sites offering sexually explicit images, what is certain is that even a casual browsing of the internet will show that such sites are numerous, offer incredibly varied content, and are easily accessed if one has the means and the inclination to do so.

None of this would surprise the men who are the subjects of this chapter, all of whom told me that it was the very ease with which they could access porn sites that was part of their problem. Most of these men had computers and smart phones for work in both their offices and their homes, so that the computers or phones themselves became a reminder of and stimulus for their sexual fantasies, not just a way of mediating and presenting them. In a sense, the sexual material on the internet had become a collective preconscious for these men. It was 'preconscious' in the sense that unlike truly repressed or unconscious material, it could easily and readily, at the flick of a computer screen, be brought into their awareness and focused perceptions, once their attention had been turned to it. And it was 'collective' in the sense that much of what the men found there was not of their own making, yet parts of it were nevertheless deeply resonant with many of their own desires.

This combination of ease of access along with the sense of certainty many of the men developed that they would always be able to find exactly the kinds of images they were looking for – as if the internet 'knew' them somehow and was providing for their wants and needs – was the primary reason men had such a difficult time abstaining from porn sites once they had decided that they must or should stop viewing them. Men found the alluring aspects of such sites to be very strong and with immediate rewards, while they could, in the short run at least, fairly easily ignore or avoid some of the more negative consequences of their browsing, such as the trouble it could and did lead to in their intimate relationships or the loss of time and energy they might have devoted to other activities. While all the men I worked with were embarrassed about spending as much time on porn sites as they did, and thought that they should hold themselves accountable for their own behaviour, several did imply that they thought their own responsibility was mitigated by the fact that the porn sites were somehow taking advantage of them and playing to their weaknesses and vulnerabilities, the very vulnerabilities and desires that Freud would have considered a core aspect of their humanness.

I should underscore again that the guilt and embarrassment these men experienced about their porn viewing was not because they were prudish or thought sex or sexual activities were somehow morally or religiously wrong. Rather, it was because they had come to realize that such repetitive viewing was putting them at risk in various ways, especially in regard to their relationships with other people, and that it had a number of dysphoric effects on them, including the sense that they were losing control of their ability to control their own behaviours and fantasies.

Freedom to Browse

While all the men I am discussing here talked openly about how much stimulation and pleasure they got from browsing porn sites – once the topic had been broached – they were only able to browse as frequently as they did because their social and economic standing afforded them access to computers or phones that could be used in relatively private contexts and for relatively private, personal reasons. All of the men held at least undergraduate degrees, several of them had more advanced education, and all of them were middle class. Almost all of these men also had jobs that allowed them to work at home or that provided them with a private office and with a computer that was dedicated to their own personal work and use, or that allowed them to use their privately owned computers and phones for work at the office. Many of the men, including one of the two I discuss at more length in the next section, also happened to live alone at the time I was seeing them, and those who lived with others had access to private bedrooms or offices where they had internet access and could browse porn sites without fear of being caught or interrupted by someone. All of the men were more comfortable viewing porn sites in the privacy of their homes because the risks of being caught at work were usually much higher than those at home. But most also reported occasional browsing at work, even if that meant taking special precautions to make sure they were not caught, including making certain that they left behind no evidence of their browsing.

I emphasize the social and economic privilege of internet access and privacy here because browsing the internet for porn is the kind of activity that can only be done with internet access and usually only in privacy, at least among the middle-class men I discuss here. While explicit forms and representations of sexuality are becoming more and more common and more accepted in all forms of media and popular culture in the United States and elsewhere in the world, all of the men I worked with would have been embarrassed for others to know how much time they spent watching porn, just as they were initially embarrassed for me to know. They were embarrassed for several reasons: one was the concern that others might think they could not get sex any other way. Another was the concern that others would judge, criticize or ridicule the kinds of bodies or sexual activities and practices they were drawn to and watching. And the men who were involved in intimate relationships of one kind or another were often concerned that if their partners knew about their browsing, these partners would feel sexually diminished, devalued or unappreciated in some way. It was the privilege of internet access and of privacy, made possible by money and education, that allowed these men to access and use internet porn in the way they did.

As I have alluded to above, most of the men eventually came to think of this privileged access to the internet and to porn as double edged. On the one hand, it allowed them to indulge and develop their sexual fantasies in ways that brought them intense and immediate pleasure. It also allowed them to express a defiant and rebellious side to themselves that they found difficult or impossible to express otherwise. But on the other hand, it also enabled them to explore and indulge their fantasies so easily and readily that most found it difficult to abstain from porn even when they were highly motivated to refrain.

I should add that none of these men consciously thought of themselves as privileged in the way I am using the term here, and they certainly did not consciously think of their access to porn as being a special benefit of their privilege or social standing. Rather, they were taking what I am calling their privileged access for granted, in much the way privileged people take their relatively good health for granted, not recognizing that good health is correlated with income, access to health insurance and medical services, location of residence and so on. Privileged, relatively risk-free access to the internet was a part of the configuration of factors contributing to how these men used internet porn and how it affected their lives, but it was also the part that was least transparent to the men themselves. They might complain that the internet made it too easy for them to indulge their fantasies, but they generally did not realize that this was a 'problem' that many other people might not have, especially those who might wish to view porn, or more porn, but whose social and economic circumstances do not allow ready access to it.

Family Histories of Conflict and Trauma and Uses of Internet Porn

The susceptibility to internet porn that I am discussing in this chapter could not have developed if the men had not had strong sexual desires and fantasies and if they had not had the kind of access to the internet that allowed them to explore their sexual fantasies fairly freely and frequently. But in the sample of men I have worked with, it is also highly correlated with a history of family conflict or trauma, a history that profoundly affected the development of their erotic lives and the particular ways in which they became attracted to and used internet porn. None of the men I worked with, for example, browsed porn sites randomly or out of boredom or mere curiosity, as many other people do. They browsed with a particular interest in mind, one that could be clearly related to earlier life events and experiences, even if the focus of that interest only became clear to them over time, as they found themselves attracted to a certain set of images repeatedly. This is important because as I noted at the outset, although all of these men were at various times intensely attracted to internet porn, and though all of them at various times felt haunted by the porn they watched – in the sense that they could not get its images out of their minds once they had viewed it and were strongly tempted to view the images repeatedly[4] – they each searched out different kinds of images and interacted with those images and fantasies in different ways.

This is a key characteristic of the complex, dynamic and multi-layered contagion-like process I am attempting to capture here: while all of the men, at one level, are being affected by porn in a similar way – they experience it as being both seductive and contaminating at the same time – at another level, from a more phenomenological perspective, they are picking up, responding to and receiving different experiences from the internet. And they in turn, with their own particular kinds of viewings and interactions, are affecting, in subtle and not so subtle ways, the reservoir of images available to anyone else accessing these porn sites. At the level of individual men, there is no single phenomenon or message being communicated and no single phenomenon or message being received. Something is actually spreading and emerging with real effects through this porn viewing process, as Gron and Meinert (2017) have suggested about social contagions in general, but the boundaries between who or what is being affected and who or what is doing the affecting are blurred, dynamically interrelated and never stable, which is likely true of all contagion-like phenomena (Hollan 2017). Indeed, one of the benefits of the 'configuring' concept is that by highlighting and foregrounding a set of dynamically interrelated factors in the development of social contagions, it underscores the dynamism and temporality of the configuration itself, the fact that we can expect social contagions to dissipate and end as well as to grow and expand.

Let me now turn to a more detailed discussion of how two of the men I am writing about actually used and interacted with internet porn sites. As we will see, both men, and most of the others who inform this chapter, had histories of anxiety and depression that they consciously related to their experiences growing up, but neither ever claimed that such experiences ever 'caused' their anxiety and depression or that their anxiety and depression ever 'caused' them to watch internet porn. Conversely, neither ever claimed that watching internet porn 'caused' their anxiety or depression. Both men had a sense that though they could be deeply affected by people and experiences, none of those isolated people or experiences ever 'caused' them to be one way rather than another, in a deterministic way. They understood that whatever their responses to these pathic influences had been, they were not straightforward or transparent, they could not have been predicted in advance, and that their effects, whatever they had been in the moment, could change over time. Both could see that their emotional states and their viewing of porn were entangled in some way, but in a way that was not easily discernible, and in a way that was likely mutually reinforcing. Indeed, mutually reinforcing enough that both men also had a sense that if they wanted their emotional states to change or improve, they would likely need to change their porn viewing habits as well.

Let me begin with Steve, a white, a-religious, middle-class professional in his forties who initially complained of depression and very intense social and interpersonal anxiety stemming at least in part, he thought, from a conflict-ridden entanglement with his parents, parents who were also socially anxious and isolated and who both struggled with their own mental health issues. Early on in our work together, we spent much time talking about Steve's problems at work, where he had fairly frequent disagreements with managers whom he considered to be overly rigid and uncreative in their supervision of his work, and from whom he felt he did not receive enough respect. We also talked at length of his attempts to find and date women, especially women who were small and petite. Initially, Steve's preference for small, slim women seemed just that, a preference, the kind of preference that many people have when thinking about the kind of person or body type they are attracted to most powerfully. But as we began to talk more extensively about his sexual interests and fantasies, Steve eventually revealed that for a very long time, he had been browsing porn sites to find images of exactly the kind of small, slim women he had been expressing a preference for. In fact, his collection of images had become so large that he spent many hours organizing and cataloguing it, to make certain that he could retrieve particular images when he wished to.

When I first asked Steve why he seemed to be so attracted to small, slim women, he could not say. He knew he liked and desired this type of woman, but beyond that, he was uncertain. As we continued to talk about this over the months, however, Steve began having dreams in which images of small, slim women would co-occur or blend with images of his neighbour as she looked when she was just reaching puberty. He then began recalling the awkwardness, shyness and inhibition of his own puberty and early adulthood. How riven he had been with sexual desire, but also how completely despairing that he would ever find someone to love or be loved by.

It was during this adolescent period that he developed an extreme crush on one of his neighbours, the one girl in his very limited social world with whom he felt safe and secure and to whom he could imagine expressing himself sexually and emotionally. As this girl neared puberty, he remembered how he would pine for the chance to catch a glimpse of some part of her exposed body. Eventually his longing became so strong that he attempted to engage the girl in sexual play, was caught by his mother, and lived for many years with the fear and dread that his mother would follow through with her threat to tell his father about his attempts at sexual play, a threat that the mother knew terrified Steve, given his father's bad temper and the father's tendency to judge people harshly for what he considered to be their 'bad' or immoral behaviour.

None of these memories about his desires for and interactions with this neighbour girl had been repressed in the classical sense. Steve had conscious access to all of them, though he had been fairly successful in suppressing and avoiding them over the intervening years. But once he began dreaming about the girl, the avoidance strategies began to break down and the memories came flooding back. As we talked about these dreams and memories, Steve eventually came to think that he had become strongly attracted to images of young, slender, petite women because their bodies reminded him, at the implicit level, of his pubescent neighbour, with whom he had had this first, though forbidden and unsuccessful, eroticized relationship. The images were allowing him to fulfil in fantasy and imagination what he had not been able to obtain as an adolescent, and they were strongly influencing what he imagined he wanted in a current sexual partner. The images did not 'cause' or initiate Steve's preoccupation with small, petite women, but they were reinforcing that preoccupation enough that Steve was beginning to realize their interconnection and beginning to understand that if he wanted to broaden the range of potential romantic partners for himself, he was also going to have to change his viewing habits.

Sociologically speaking, Ted was similar to Steve. He too was a white, a-religious, middle-class professional in his thirties. Unlike Steve, however, Ted came into therapy because he and his live-in girlfriend of several years had been having relationship problems. Although Ted was a member of a twelve-step programme and was worried that he had inherited his father's depression, he also was concerned that he was no longer sexually attracted to his girlfriend, and so had become highly ambivalent about marrying her. We talked for several months about his depressive feelings, his obsession with work and his lack of sexual interest in his girlfriend before he was able and willing to tell me about his frequent visits to dominatrixes and his even more frequent browsing of dominatrix sites on the internet.

In some ways, this revelation was not a surprise to me. Ted, though a physically large man, came across as a 'small' person – earnest, quiet, self-contained, self-effacing and deferential. His interpersonal style was to lie low and avoid conflict by 'submitting' himself to others – as he learned to do around his abusive father, a man who eventually became diagnosed with a serious mental disorder, drank heavily, and terrified the family with his temper and erratic behaviour. Ted told me that he spent many hours as a youth both before and after school attempting to avoid his father by hiding out in his own room. Things were bad enough, he said, that he eventually came to develop the strong conviction that his father would one day shoot and kill the whole family and then shoot and kill himself.

Like Steve, Ted was highly selective about the internet sites he browsed, despite the nearly limitless supply and variety of sexual stimulation and fantasy that is readily available on the web. He was particularly drawn to the sites of beautiful, dramatically dressed dominatrixes who posted fictional or non-fictional accounts of their clients' fantasies and adventures. When he found stories that resonated with his own sexual fantasies and/or excited him sexually, he was more likely to return to a site, and more likely, eventually, to contact its proprietor to schedule an in-person session. When Ted *did* return to a site to schedule a session, he would often email his own fantasy story in advance, so that the dominatrix knew exactly what to do to stimulate and satisfy him. On occasion, Ted's own activities and fantasies ended up being posted on a site, which then attracted (or not) the interest of other browsers.

Many of Ted's dominatrix fantasies and behaviours tended to recreate and reflect, in exaggerated and dramatic fashion, his past family experiences and his reactions to them: the danger, the humiliation, the sense of unworthiness and powerlessness, all fused with sexual arousal – one of the few, if secret, activities of his youth that brought him pleasure and self-soothing. He submitted himself to the denigration and beatings of the dominatrixes, but in return, their beauty and power stimulated him sexually. He submitted so that eventually he could triumph, if only in privacy and if only in fantasy.[5]

Unlike Steve, however, Ted himself had little conscious insight into how or why these fantasies and proclivities had developed: he knew that he enjoyed being with and fantasizing about dominatrixes and that the women he consorted with either as an in-person client or in fantasy were always prettier and sexier than his actual girlfriend or other women he thought he could realistically date. He knew that he enjoyed the risk-taking and the beatings because they were, he said, like 'shock treatments' that 'jump started' him physically. And he knew that these impulsive, flamboyant and emotionally charged activities were the antithesis of his everyday behaviours, which, as I mentioned, were characterized by a rather narrow and concentrated focus on work, the sense of feeling empty inside, and by an avoidant, deferential interpersonal style. Yet he could not readily see or understand how these two sides of himself were related, as scholars and researchers of dissociation might hypothesize (Bromberg 1998; Stern 1997; Stoler 1975; Van der Kolk 2014).

Ted was somewhat less shame-ridden than Steve about his porn interests, largely because up until the time we worked together, no one had even suspected that he might have the kind of sexual interests and fantasies he did, much less catch him actually indulging in those fantasies. Indeed, Ted would occasionally wonder what his chances were of meeting a woman in his day-to-day life who might share his sexual interests. Yet he was also aware that his sexual fantasies and activities were putting him at risk of exposure to colleagues, friends and family, including his girlfriend, and that they were costing him a lot of money. So Ted too, at the end of the day, was hoping that he could spend less time on the internet and with his dominatrix partners.

An important feature of both cases is the link between porn viewing and feelings of depression and social isolation. Long before either man had started viewing porn, each had grown up feeling unsafe and unhappy at home, which in turn had led to each feeling insecure and mistrustful in many social situations, especially those involving intimacy or sexuality. By the time both men were old enough to have access to the internet, both had become socially isolated, and both were beginning to find it easier to explore their sexual identities and fantasies online rather than with other people in their day-to-day lives, which is another way in which they differ from others who view porn. As both men told me, internet porn was not 'causing' this social isolation – no one or thing was forcing them to watch – but its ease of access was enabling them to escape the anxiety of working out their sexuality with actual partners, and was doing so in such a way as to reinforce fantasies carried over from their troubled youths, by allowing them to so easily find images tailor-made to those fantasies. This was the aspect of their viewing that made it obsessive-like and this was the aspect that most distinguishes these men from many others who watch porn more casually and without the sense of being haunted by it.

Concluding Thoughts: Internet Porn and Social Contagion

It is not an exaggeration to say that internet porn is everywhere these days. Turn on a computer almost anywhere in the world, and if you have the inclination, you can find sexually explicit images of almost any kind. Through its mediating role, the internet has exposed countless numbers of people to the kinds of sexual images and practices that many of them have likely only dreamed or fantasized about, if that, in the same way that it has exposed countless people to, and made readily available, many other types of knowledge, images, artefacts and experiences. To that extent, the internet is a prime vector and facilitator of many types of social contagion, including porn.

While the spreading of porn around the world can itself be seen as a type of contagion, my concern in this chapter is on a subset of all those exposed to porn, those who view it fairly frequently and those who are 'haunted' by their exposure in the sense that they cannot stop watching, even when they wish to refrain, and in the sense that their viewing habits interfere, either directly or indirectly, with their attempts to develop and maintain offline intimate and sexual relationships. Although the people whom I discuss in this chapter are all male and heterosexual, I have every reason to believe that the configuration of vectors and variables that contribute to these men being especially vulnerable to the haunting effects of porn would affect others in a similar way, no matter what their gender or sexual preference. Assuming for the moment, along with Freud, that all humans eventually develop sexual fantasies, it is the history of family conflict and resulting social mistrust and isolation, coupled with 'privileged' access to the internet, that configure the susceptibility to porn that I have described in this chapter. Because many people other than male heterosexuals have privileged access to the internet and come from backgrounds of family conflict, I suspect that many others may be 'haunted' by porn in the ways I have described here, though because porn viewing is often/usually conducted in solitude or relative privacy, the actual numbers are difficult to investigate. Of course, viewing porn in solitude or relative privacy may itself lead or contribute to social isolation and depressive-like feelings, but if such viewing does not resonate deeply with sexual fantasies left over from earlier life experiences, I suggest that it is less likely to develop the kind of obsessive, repetitive-like qualities that were characteristic of the way Steve and Ted viewed porn.

An important aspect of this 'contagion' is that while all the men I have discussed were susceptible to porn and were deeply affected by it, they were susceptible in their own particular ways. None of the men viewed or consumed even a fraction of the vast reservoir of sexually explicit images that are available on the internet, even though that vast reservoir, which I have likened to a collective preconscious, was readily available to them. Rather, their browsing was much more selective, either consciously or unconsciously related to sexual fantasies that had originally developed in an earlier period of life. Steve's attraction to images of small, slim, petite women was consciously related to the erotic relationship he had developed to a neighbouring girl as a young adolescent, while Ted's preoccupation with dominatrixes was unconsciously related to the danger and humiliation he had experienced growing up with a troubled and abusive father. Steve and Ted were both dipping into the reservoir of sexual images commonly available to both of them, but in different places, and in both cases that dipping was reinforcing fantasies left over from an earlier period of life, but fantasies of a very different nature. The contagious element here – internet porn – was gaining access to these imaginatively different 'hosts' by offering images that were selectively and differentially attractive to them, demonstrating not only that the thing being spread in a social contagion might be non-unitary and polysemous, but also the messages or experiences being received (Hollan 2017). For the cases being discussed here, one person's 'porn' was clearly not another person's porn.

But if the contagious images were gaining access and affecting people in different ways, it is equally interesting that people's viewing habits, in turn, were affecting and reshaping the collective reservoir of sexually explicit images that were available to others. Selective browsing leads to the 'thickening', or to the increasing numbers and diversification, of content that is selected for and to the pruning of content that is not. By selectively and frequently browsing certain websites and not others, Steve and Ted were both contributing to this process and were affecting the kinds of images that others might come across as they browse for porn, casually or otherwise. Ted contributed to this process in more direct ways as well, by offering his sexual fantasies to certain dominatrixes whom he knew would post them for others to see and be stimulated by. This selective presentation of highly personalized ideas and fantasies into a more public arena for others to either pick up on and further transform and elaborate or not, and the reverse, the use of publicly available images to help express and articulate highly personal ideas and fantasies (or not), is characteristic of the social and cultural process as a whole, according to someone like Obeyesekere (1981, 1990). And if so, then we see that social contagions of any kind, whether of porn or anything else, are merely special cases of how social processes and influences work more broadly, though usually in a more accelerated and visible fashion: partially, incrementally, in a 'condensed' way, through a variety of sensory and perceptual modalities, contingent on and delimited by the emotional memories of those involved, but with the potential of exceeding those contingencies and limitations by the ability of all of the participants to imaginatively elaborate upon what is experienced and communicated (Hollan 2017). All people are affected by others and material substances, but selectively, in ways that are often less direct and obvious than many people would suspect. And all people affect others and material substances, though again in ways that are often less obvious and direct than usually supposed. In the cases I have discussed here, this selectivity is enabled and constrained not only by technology and socioeconomic class, but by the experiential residues of men's past social encounters.

The complexity and dynamism of the contagion-like processes I have sketched here raises the issue of their boundaries with other types of social processes. When, where, and by whom or what do they actually start? When, where, and by whom or what do they actually end? Who or what is particularly susceptible to a certain kind of social contagion and who or what is not? A key benefit of the configuring concept is that it captures and highlights this complexity and dynamism, first, by emphasizing that all contagions are temporal processes and so in dynamic flux or stasis subject to change; and second, by noting that the vectors and variables contributing to the configuration of a social contagion are themselves likely to change with time, so that they are subject to falling into or out of a given configuration and to interacting with other elements of the configuration in new ways, resulting in either the intensification of a contagion or its dissipation.

In the case of the men I have discussed here, the most constant element of the configuration of factors leading to their haunting by porn was the fact that they likely would have fantasized about sex under any conditions we could imagine. Their privileged access to computers and the internet was more subject to change, though, and several of the men who inform this chapter were badly affected by the severe economic recession beginning in 2007–08, losing incomes and jobs, which did make it more difficult for some of them to access porn as frequently as they had before. None of the men could change their family histories of conflict or trauma that correlate so strongly with some of their most core sexual and erotic fantasies, of course, but because all of them had sought out therapy, they all had the potential of reworking their emotional reactions to those histories and the susceptibility to obsessive-like porn viewing that came with them, and several of them did. But this access to therapy was also affected by the recession of 2007–08, and some of the men had to give up therapy before their potential for emotional and erotic change could be realized through a therapeutic process. And no doubt some of these men, over time, would be lucky enough or fortunate enough to discover non-porn ways of addressing their core sexual fantasies, as Ted was hoping to find a partner who would join with him in his dominatrix fantasies, or would experience those fantasies changing through other types of experiences in their lives, whether positive or negative. My point here, again, is that any configuration of factors leading to the development of a social contagion is always in a state of dynamic flux and subject to change, whether obvious from a third person point of view or not.

Finally, although many clinicians and mental health scholars would now disagree with Freud's contention that conflicts over sexuality and eroticism form the core of many, if not most, mental and emotional disorders, the material I have presented here does remind us that Freud and other psychoanalysts are certainly right in suggesting that sexuality and eroticism are always implicated in emotional life and social experience, if not as cause, then as consequence. Although both Steve and Ted had serious problems not directly related to their sexuality (depression and anxiety, drug use, history of family conflict and trauma, impaired self-esteem), their sexual and erotic lives were certainly directly affected by these other problems, and with the social processes in which they were entangled. This is an aspect of social and emotional experience that comes to the fore when we focus on how porn viewing is implicated in people's lives, but of course it is an important aspect of *all* social experience, including all social contagions, and one that is certainly worthy of more focused attention and analysis.

Douglas Hollan
Professor and Luckman Distinguished Teacher
Department of Anthropology, University of California, Los Angeles

Notes

1. In addition to being an anthropologist, I have clinical training in psychoanalysis and I am licensed by the state of California as a 'research psychoanalyst'. The analyses I have conducted are for both therapeutic and research purposes, and as such, the identities of the people I write about are always disguised and altered to protect anonymity.
2. Four or five of my analyses with heterosexual men immediately come to mind. Though the absolute numbers are small, they reflect a surprisingly high percentage of the men I have worked with over the years, and the pattern of first hiding the viewing of internet porn and then revealing it only after a great deal of therapeutic trust has been built up is very striking and suggestive. Indeed, this leads me to think that far more people are

haunted by internet porn than ever come to light in psychoanalysis or elsewhere.
3. For a recent survey and discussion of the philosophical literature on imagination and the imaginary, including contributions from psychoanalysis, see Lennon (2015).
4. Note that I use 'haunted' is its colloquial sense, to indicate how an image, thought, feeling, emotion or other phenomenon may be difficult to rid from one's consciousness. This is related to, but different from, the more formal study of 'hauntology' as defined by Derrida (1994), Gordon (2008), Good (2015, this volume) or Hollan (2019).
5. For a more detailed discussion of this case, see Hollan (2004).

References

Bromberg, Phillip. 1998. *Standing in the Spaces: Essays on Clinical Process, Trauma, and Dissociation*. Hillsdale, NJ: Analytic Press.

Caughey, John. 1984. *Imaginary Social Worlds: A Cultural Approach*. Lincoln: University of Nebraska Press.

Derrida, Jacques. 1994. *Specters of Marx: The State of the Debt, the Work of Mourning, and the New International*. New York: Routledge.

Dilley, R.M. 1999. 'Introduction', in R.M. Dilley (ed.), *The Problem of Context: Perspectives from Social Anthropology and Elsewhere*. New York: Berghahn Books.

Freud, Sigmund. 2010. *Civilization and Its Discontents*. New York: W.W. Norton.

Gammeltoft, Tine M. 2014. 'Toward an Anthropology of the Imaginary: Specters of Disability in Vietnam', *Ethos* 42: 153–74.

Good, Byron J. 2015. 'Haunted by Aceh: Specters of Violence in Post-Suharto Indonesia', in Devon E. Hinton and Alexander L. Hinton (eds), *Genocide and Mass Violence: Memory, Symptom, and Recovery*. Cambridge: Cambridge University Press, pp. 58–82.

Gordon, Avery. 2008. *Ghostly Matters: Haunting and the Sociological Imagination*. Minneapolis: University of Minnesota Press.

Gron, Lone, and Lotte Meinert. 2017. 'Social Contagion and Cultural Epidemics: Phenomenological and "Experience-Near" Explorations', *Ethos* 45(2): 165–81.

Hollan, Douglas. 2004. 'Self Systems, Cultural Idioms of Distress, and the Psycho-Bodily Consequences of Childhood Illness', *Transcultural Psychiatry* 41(1): 62–79.

———. 2017. 'Dreamscapes of Intimacy and Isolation: Shadows of Contagion and Immunity', *Ethos* 45(2): 216–31.

———. 2019. 'Who Is Haunted by Whom? Steps to an Ecology of Haunting', *Ethos* 47: 451–64.

Isaacs, Susan. 1952. 'The Nature and Function of Fantasy', in Joan Riviere (ed.), *Developments in Psycho-Analysis*. London: Hogarth Press, pp. 67–121.

Klein, Melanie. 1964. *Contributions to Psychoanalysis, 1921–1945*. New York: McGraw-Hill.

——. 1975. *Envy and Gratitude and Other Works, 1946–1963*. New York: Delacorte Press.

Lennon, Kathleen. 2015. *Imagination and the Imaginary*. New York: Routledge.

Lindholm, Charles. 2001. *Culture and Identity: The History, Theory, and Practice of Psychological Anthropology*. New York: McGraw-Hill.

Obeyesekere, Gananath. 1981. *Medusa's Hair: An Essay on Personal Symbols and Religious Experience*. Chicago: University of Chicago Press.

——. 1990. *The Work of Culture: Symbolic Transformation in Psychoanalysis and Anthropology*. Chicago: University of Chicago Press.

Seeberg, Jens, and Lotte Meinert. 2015. 'Can Epidemics Be Non-Communicable? Reflections on the Spread of "Non-Communicable Diseases"', *Medicine Anthropology Theory* 2(2): 54–71.

Stern, Daniel. 1997. *Unformulated Experience: From Dissociation to Imagination in Psychoanalysis*. Hillsdale, NY: Analytic Press.

Stoler, Robert. 1975. *Perversions*. New York: Pantheon.

Van der Kolk, Bessel. 2014: *The Body Keeps the Score: Brain, Mind, and Body in the Healing of Trauma*. New York: Penguin Group.

Chapter 9
Contagious Configurations
Reproductive Governance from Abortion to Zika Virus in Latin America

Lynn M. Morgan

Introduction

In late 2015, Brazil reported an increase in the incidence of microcephaly[1] in newborns, thought to be associated with an epidemic of mosquito-borne Zika virus. On 1 February 2016, the World Health Organization (WHO) labelled the epidemic a Public Health Emergency of International Concern (PHEIC), after the effects of congenital Zika syndrome were definitively linked to the Zika virus. The Pan American Health Organization (PAHO), the regional branch of the WHO for the Americas, responded with education and prevention campaigns that focused mainly on controlling the *Aedes aegypti* mosquito. Along with the US-based Centers for Disease Control and Prevention (CDC) and regional governments,[2] PAHO issued travel advisories to warn women who were pregnant or planning to become pregnant to avoid travel to affected areas. Some government officials suggested that women avoid becoming pregnant as long as Zika virus was present. Even after Zika was recognized as a sexually transmitted infection, health authorities hesitated to recommend contraceptive methods (especially condoms) or prenatal screening, nor did they mount campaigns to inform women about pregnancy termination options even in locations where abortion was legal. By November 2016, with forty-seven countries and territories in the Americas reporting Zika outbreaks over the previous twelve months,[3] 'no national or international health organization has issued any guidance on the reproductive options that should be available to women where Zika transmission remains a risk' (Fernandes 2017).

In this chapter, I argue that our efforts to 'configure contagion' must take account of the politics that affect how a multilateral agency such as PAHO conceptualizes and addresses social suffering. No epidemic spreads unmitigated by social and political forces, as the chapters in this volume attest. The spread of Zika virus is affected by 'climate variation, land-use change, poverty, and human movement' (S. Ali et al. 2017), but also by politics. Here I argue that PAHO, as the principal international health governance body in the western hemisphere, violated its own long-standing commitment to rights-based public health by ignoring the reproductive health dimensions of Zika virus in its initial response to the outbreak. PAHO amplified certain forms of technocratic knowledge (such as mosquito control and vaccine development) while ignoring those that required attention to gender equity, contraception, pregnancy management and services for neurologically disabled children. By taking an ostensibly apolitical approach, PAHO 'configured contagion' in ways that were narrowly technocratic and conservative. PAHO's conspicuous inattention to the reproductive health dimensions of the crisis violated its own commitment to working closely within the Inter-American human rights system. PAHO was complicit in perpetuating ignorance, amplifying suffering and ensuring that the worst consequences of the epidemic would be borne by low-income women who lack access to education, medical care and social services for disabled children.

PAHO's configuration of contagion in the Zika epidemic was cautious to the point of being cowardly. Just as epidemics spread through contagion, so too do ideas about who is most at risk and what actions governmental agencies can take to prevent or treat them. When a multilateral organization such as PAHO overlooks an opportunity to educate people about sexual transmission of the virus, or to offer enhanced access to contraception or abortion to those at risk, it ensures that the virus will disproportionately affect women and the poor. By censoring itself over topics it deemed controversial, PAHO ensured that certain aspects of Zika transmission related to sexuality and reproduction would be literally non-communicable, that is, unable to be communicated via civil or public health discourse. PAHO's configuration of contagion in the Zika epidemic shows how the agency engaged in a kind of reproductive governance that naturalized sacrifice and suffering on the part of people who were poor, pregnant and potentially pregnant. By ignoring the need to expand access to contraception and abortion during the epidemic, it created a 'generation Zika' (Hodge 2016) and perpetuated a pattern of reproductive governance that ignores the social and political rights of women and the poor.

The concept of reproductive governance relies on a combination of Foucauldian poststructuralism and political-economic critique to show how rights-bearing subjects (microcephalic infants and their mothers, for example) are created, managed and subjected to state surveillance (Morgan and Roberts 2012). It shows how Zika-afflicted women and children are incorporated into public discourse, how states represent gendered sexual morality and how reproduction figures in contexts of neoliberal restructuring. Even as the world's first Latin American pope expressed compassion towards parishioners in Zika-affected regions who might wish to practise contraception, PAHO did not encourage local governments to expand access to sexual health education, contraception or therapeutic abortion. PAHO therefore failed to 'mainstream' its own rights-based, secular and gender-sensitive policies, choosing instead to side with the conservative religious activists working to thwart the advance of sexual and reproductive rights. These conservatives seem to have exerted a 'contagious' authority that infected public health governance, concealed certain treatment options and policy responses and kept authorities from venturing to offer comprehensive reproductive health services.

The concept of contagion extends beyond the spread of arboviruses, their vectors, infected persons and their caretakers to include the culture of the policymakers who managed the Zika outbreak. This biosocial configuration determines the contours of the ongoing epidemic: who will be affected, where resources will (and will not) be directed and whether Zika virus will be used to incorporate reproductive rights into its ostensibly rights-based approach to public health. The current configuration perpetuates abortion stigma and secrecy by avoiding any mention of pregnancy termination or recommending changes in abortion access laws and protocols (Kumar, Hessini and Mitchell 2009). Such political cowardice reflects an abdication of the responsibility to implement international human rights laws and standards regarding reproductive health, rights and justice.

Disputes over Abortion and the Reproductive Health Implications of the Zika Epidemic

As soon as the devastating effects on foetal health became apparent, Zika was transformed into another flashpoint in the ongoing debate over abortion rights in the Americas. In 2012, Brazil had made abortion legal in cases of anencephaly, but the law would not apply to cases of microcephaly. Abortion is completely prohibited in some of the countries hard hit by Zika: Nicaragua, El Salvador, Honduras and the Dominican Republic (Langer, Caglia and Menéndez 2016: 180). Yet the global governance bodies are presumably acting above the ideological and legal constraints imposed by nation-states. As sovereign bodies made up of member states, they arguably have greater latitude to act in the public interest and in the interest of public health. At the United Nations in February 2016, the High Commissioner for Human Rights advised Latin American countries affected by the Zika virus to legalize abortion, so that pregnant women in affected regions could choose whether to continue their pregnancies. The WHO was not as bold. It issued conflicting advice, first advising women to delay pregnancy in Zika-affected zones, then recommending that people should be 'offered contraception and counselling to help decide whether to become pregnant' (McNeil 2016). Members of the Emergency Committee convened by WHO to offer suggestions about managing the epidemic were loath to be specific about abortion, suggesting only 'guidance to be available to pregnant women so that they better understand the present situation and are empowered to make a decision about personal protection and pregnancy' (Heymann et al. 2016).

The debate over the relationship between Zika and abortion quickly polarized along familiar lines, with Latin American women's health and reproductive rights advocates arguing that this epidemic was another in a series (rubella, HIV/AIDS) showing how women are denied the right to choose their own reproductive futures. Women would ideally be supported through neutral, unbiased counselling about their reproductive options, whether they decided to terminate a pregnancy or 'carry the pregnancy to term, with full social support' (Carmago 2016: 3; see also Adams 2016; Diniz 2016a, 2016b; Roa 2016). On the other end of the political spectrum, Catholic and pro-life activists argued that abortion rights advocates were exploiting the epidemic 'to promote the legalization of abortion-on-demand throughout Latin America' (CitizenGO 2016). One argued that abortion was a costly 'distraction' from addressing the need for basic preventive health care and vaccine development (de Campos 2016), while another interpreted the epidemiological data as evidence that a 'false alarm' over Zika had led to 'untold unnecessary abortions' (Garcia Jones 2016). In Brazil, anti-choice legislators introduced a bill proposing to 'increase jail time for abortions carried out *"due to microcephaly or other foetal anomaly"'* (Camargo 2016: 1; emphasis in original). In the United States, the Republican-controlled Congress held up then-President Barack Obama's request for a $1.1 billion funding appropriation in September 2016, proposing to allocate the funds only if Planned Parenthood were exempted from the recipient list (Huetteman and Tavernise 2016; see also Hodge 2016: 41).

Abortion politics have been a central subtext in government responses to the Zika epidemic. El Salvador advised women not to become pregnant for two years, even though abortion has been banned there since 1998 and contraceptive methods can be difficult to obtain. Such recommendations were widely criticized by feminist health advocates who note that women are not allowed to control their reproductive lives (González and Diniz 2016). As Joshua Krisch (2016) wrote, 'The irony, which seems lost on El Salvador, is that the same government that denies women control over their reproductive health is now asking those same women to control their reproductive health until 2018'. The urgency of the situation makes it even more striking that PAHO authorities declined to suggest or even mention abortion, apparently for fear of inciting religious conservatives (McNeil 2017). Even in places where abortion is legal, such as the United States, the CDC did not, as of August 2019, mention the possibility of pregnancy termination as an option for pregnant women who are infected with the Zika virus (Goldthwaite and Velasquez 2016: 501).

PAHO is obligated by its own policy guidelines to respect the laws and sovereignty of member nations, which explains why it might hesitate to issue recommendations that challenge those laws. Still, PAHO remained relatively silent even when it could have taken a leadership role to emphasize the public health urgency of providing access to comprehensive reproductive health counselling and services. The burden of its reticence is shouldered by pregnant women who live in affected regions. Because there is no easy test for Zika infection and 80 per cent of cases are asymptomatic, it is almost impossible for pregnant women to know whether they or their foetuses are afflicted. Those who live in affected areas do not benefit from travel bans. This leads to high levels of anxiety among pregnant women living in the Zika zones. In the absence of concrete information, some undoubtedly terminate their pregnancies clandestinely rather than risk having a child with severe neurological defects. Untold numbers of women in Zika-affected Colombia were apparently worried enough about the potential danger to their foetuses that they terminated their pregnancies even without the benefit of medical attention, thus reducing the incidence of microcephaly there (Aiken et al. 2016; McNeil and Cobb 2016). They may have felt compelled to do so knowing that they would have little access to 'effective medical and social services for handicapped children' given that they live in poverty (Fernandes 2017). The conspiracy of silence inhibits our ability to collect accurate information about how women are managing pregnancy in Zika-afflicted zones. 'Anecdotal evidence suggests more women have been quietly terminating pregnancies over worries that their babies might be deformed' (Phillips and Miroff 2016). Meanwhile, 2,700 children in the western hemisphere were confirmed to have congenital syndrome associated with Zika virus as of 9 February 2017. Although PAHO could have used the Zika outbreak to promote pregnancy termination options, it did not do so. Abortion laws and policies remain largely unchanged in the region, suggesting that the Zika virus epidemic had no effect on reproductive health policy (Carabali et al. 2018).

A Human Rights Approach

Because WHO and PAHO have openly committed to a rights-based approach to health, several scholars argue that these agencies have an obligation to respond appropriately to the Zika epidemic using the frameworks of human rights and to encourage local governments to do the same. 'Responses to public health emergencies are the responsibility of governments', they note (Diniz et al. 2017: 106), and 'countries bear responsibility for national health plans consistent with their international human rights obligations' (Gruskin, Bogecho and Ferguson 2010: 130). Appropriate responses to a public health emergency of the type presented by the Zika epidemic would therefore include not just mosquito control efforts, but comprehensive public education campaigns (including information about the sexual transmission of the virus and access to legal abortion), ready public access to contraceptive technologies (including long-acting reversible methods such as IUDs) and the 'legal right to pregnancy termination' for 'infected pregnant women experiencing intense, health-impairing anxiety about their future and that of their children' (Diniz et al. 2017: 106; see also Ali, Miller and Gómez 2017; Gruskin, Bogecho and Ferguson 2010; Leite 2016; Roa 2016).

One of the biggest concerns expressed by feminist and human rights advocates is that governments have responded to the Zika outbreak in ways that reinforce, rather than mitigate, social stratification and gender discrimination (González and Diniz 2016). International human rights accords governing reproductive health and child welfare are especially attentive to the discriminatory effects of government policies, but governments did not invoke these accords when responding to the Zika emergency. For example, low-income women have a high unmet need for contraceptive services and prenatal care and are 'the most likely to be exposed to vector-borne illnesses' (Langer, Caglia and Menéndez 2016: 180). As a result, low-income women suffer the consequences of coping with 'hazardous pregnancies and legal constraints on termination', while wealthier women can gain access to prenatal care and abortion (including extra-legal or clandestine services) in safe conditions (Diniz 2017: 107). This disparity functions to keep abortion restrictions intact, they point out, because the policymakers are themselves wealthy enough to access private abortion when necessary and therefore feel no compulsion to loosen restrictive laws (Diniz et al. 2017: 107–8). Class inequality therefore has a gendered impact; it exposes women to structural violence including unwanted pregnancy and then denies them access to abortion, thus limiting their ability to improve their economic chances and escape from poverty (González and Diniz 2016). Throughout the Zika epidemic, feminist and women's health advocates found that they could not rely on PAHO for collaboration and were thus forced to work independently of the region's major health governing agency. This situation set up a configuration of contagion in which abortion restrictions reinforced health, economic and power disparities in a vicious cycle, keeping poor women as well as elite feminist activists from gaining further control over their sexual and reproductive futures.

PAHO is explicitly committed to a health and human rights approach that is 'firmly based on international human rights treaties' (Gruskin, Bogecho and Ferguson 2010: 135). Human rights standards are legally binding on states under domestic and international covenants, as Diniz and colleagues point out, and 'denial and obstruction of sexual and reproductive health services ... can constitute human rights violations' (2017: 107). Feminist legal scholar Paola Bergallo argues that denying legal abortion to Brazilian Zika-infected women 'is inconsistent with the commitments undertaken by Brazil in its constitution and the human rights treaties signed by the country in regard to the rights of women' (Román 2016). Rights-based approaches to health are drawn, in part, from the American Convention on Human Rights and rulings handed down through the Inter-American health rights system. If PAHO's rights-based approach were to be assessed based on its grounding in international rights law, the agency should have reacted to the Zika outbreak by emphasizing the legal standards enacted by the Inter-American Court of Human Rights (IACHR) in its landmark 2012 ruling, *Artavia Murillo et al. ('In Vitro Fertilization') v. Costa Rica*. That case called on Costa Rica to reinstate its twelve-year ban on in vitro fertilization. More importantly for our purposes, the ruling also established for the first time in international law that reproductive rights are human rights, that embryos cannot be considered juridical 'persons', and that the rights of embryos may not take precedence over those of women. The IACHR clarified Article 4.1 of the American Convention on Human Rights, stating that 'conception' should be defined not as the fertilization of gametes but as the implantation of an embryo in a woman's womb. Decisions made by the Inter-American Court are binding on the twenty-three countries that have ratified the American Convention on Human Rights. The decision establishes the right to reproductive autonomy, the right to access reproductive health services and the notion that embryos are best protected by protecting the rights of pregnant women.

PAHO has incorporated an explicit focus on human rights into its strategic health agenda for the Americas and has worked closely with the Inter-American human rights system to advance a consistent message (Meier and Ayala 2014: 364). Nevertheless, the IACHR's decision that 'reproductive rights are human rights' did not appear in PAHO's directives during the Zika outbreak. PAHO did not use Zika as an opportunity to engage in national capacity building on reproductive rights. As far as I can tell, PAHO did not disseminate information about the IACHR ruling or show how it could be related to Zika-response policies, which could have justified any government's decision to offer pregnancy termination to women concerned about the impact of the Zika virus on their foetuses. If PAHO had cited the IACHR ruling in response to the Zika outbreak, it could have reminded member nations of their obligation to comply with international law and to respect reproductive rights as a component of human rights.

The Global Gag Rule's Insensitivity to the Zika Implications

Policies formulated in the United States can have a major impact on global health policy. Democratic administrations have tended to support the language of human rights and women's rights, while Republican administrations have not. According to Meier and Ayala, there was a 'public silence on human rights issues in the early 2000s, with the United States then objecting to any mention of human rights beyond the WHO Constitution' (2014: 368). On President Donald J. Trump's fourth day in office in January 2017, he reinstated the so-called 'global gag rule', which prohibits federal funding from programmes or agencies that 'provide, promote, or make referrals to abortion services, or give information about abortions' (Singh and Karim 2017). Global health experts pointed out that this rule would affect access to contraception, HIV testing and treatment and gender-based violence reporting; it would likely result in an increased number of abortions around the world. It would in some cases require physicians and NGOs to violate the abortion laws, bill of rights and professional codes of ethics of the countries in which they work (Singh and Karim 2017: 387). It would also cut off funding for contraceptive services when provided by NGOs that also offer abortion services, which would have an adverse effect on pregnancy prevention in Zika-afflicted regions (Singh and Karim 2017: 388). As a result of the re-institutionalization of the global gag rule, one feminist health advocate said, 'We expect a blanket silence on abortion from health workers funded by the US government in all fields – not just reproductive health or family planning. For example, women receiving HIV testing and treatment or who have suffered from gender-based violence won't be informed about or referred to abortion services'.[4] This policy created a 'climate of intimidation' (Fegan and Rebouche 2003) and had a chilling effect on the willingness of PAHO officials to challenge Trump administration officials. This assault on human rights later intensified, with the United States actively attacking progressive human rights as promulgated by the United Nations, the World Health Organization and the Organization of American States. Such a cowardly attitude emboldens abortion opponents in the Americas, thus inhibiting the possibility of imminent policy shifts.

Conclusion

Feminist and women's health advocates were instrumental in insisting that Zika virus is a sexually transmitted disease that needs to be approached from a human rights perspective. In Brazil, one such group – Anis: Institute of Bioethics, Human Rights and Gender – filed suit with the Brazilian Supreme Court charging that the government must allow women in Zika-affected communities access to preventive measures as well as elective termination of pregnancy in order to avoid mental distress (Boseley 2016). Their work was vital to insisting that rights-based approaches be applied to the Zika epidemic. Without them, mainstream international health agencies such as PAHO and the CDC showed that they were disinclined to consider Zika in reproductive rights terms. The PAHO informational page about Zika and pregnancy posed – but gave only a feeble response to – the question of whether women should 'postpone or interrupt pregnancy' as a result of Zika: 'Any decision to defer pregnancy is a woman's human right. PAHO urges public health authorities to ensure that women have access to reproductive health services, including contraception, are well informed about personal protection from mosquito bites and about the eventual risks to which they may be exposed. Women should also be informed of the support services they can expect to receive after birth'. Nowhere did PAHO mention the need to provide elective termination of pregnancy, even in the event of active, diagnosed Zika infection during pregnancy.[5]

During the height of the Zika outbreak in Latin America, epidemiologists and journalists devoted most of their attention to tradition biomedical epistemologies of contagion, such as exposure to infected mosquitoes during a vulnerable stage of embryological development. Yet a more pernicious process of social contagion was unfolding simultaneously, in an epidemic of self-censorship, fear and cowardice that gripped international public health authorities and constrained their ability to respond to the epidemic. Rather than adopting a progressive, rights-based public health response, international and national public health authorities allowed themselves to be silenced by religious conservatives who objected to any public health response that might mention contraception or pregnancy termination. Indeed, religious conservatives mounted a vociferous pre-emptive campaign to keep public health authorities from mentioning reproductive health or rights. Headlines in the anti-abortion press, for example, included: 'Pregnant teen with Zika rejects abortion pressure: "God has given me a miracle"'; 'How to defeat the Zika virus without killing innocent babies'; '"In no way does this justify abortion": Pro-life leaders react to study linking Zika, microcephaly'; 'US Congress scolds UN rights chief for exploiting Zika to push abortion'; 'Top American Catholic ethics body says no to contraception for Zika'.[6] Opponents of abortion argued that Zika babies are innocent, that sacrificial mothers should take care of their sick and disabled children and that it is egotistical and wrong to interfere with God's plan. They insisted, in a dynamic and intersubjective process of social contagion, that public health authorities support (or at least not contradict) their position.

The Latin American social order has been influenced by an increasingly powerful alliance of conservative religious leaders who affect reproductive governance by wielding considerable influence over public health authorities. This case study highlights the extent to which configurations of contagion must take account of socially powerful actors, including those not directly implicated in the circulation of viral pathogens. As public health authorities in Latin America weighed their possible responses to mitigating the Zika epidemic and its dramatic consequences, they had to consider not just who would benefit from their policies, but who they could least afford to offend. Unfortunately, they mostly chose to mollify conservative religious actors rather than protecting women's rights to autonomous reproductive decision-making. This gave religious conservatives (both Catholics and evangelicals) the latitude to pressure health authorities into concealing prevention and treatment options that the conservatives found objectionable. The resulting repression of reproductive health, rights and justice resulted from a particular biosocial configuration that had a definite (albeit unmeasurable) impact on how the Zika epidemic unfolded in Latin America.

Public health authorities, including those working with PAHO, were complicit in perpetuating a cautious form of reproductive governance that violates international human rights accords as well as their own commitments to gender- and human rights mainstreaming. In the early months of the epidemic, they abdicated their responsibility to demonstrate courageous leadership, thus perpetuating a discriminatory pattern of Zika-inflicted health and gender disparities. This case study shows a 'configuration of contagion' in which social and biological factors are intertwined and fuelled by the powerful social contaminants of intimidation and fear.

Lynn M. Morgan
Professor Emerita, Department of Sociology and Anthropology
Mount Holyoke College, Massachusetts, USA

Notes

1. Now called Congenital Zika Syndrome (CZS).
2. The governments of Brazil, Colombia, El Salvador, Jamaica and Puerto Rico advised women to avoid pregnancy during the epidemic (McNeil 2016).
3. WHO, 'Countries and Territories That Have Reported Mosquito-Borne Zika Virus Transmission', retrieved 19 June 2021 from http://www.who.int/emergencies/zika-virus/situation-report/Table1_27102016.pdf?ua=1.
4. AWID, 'Feminist Standpoints on the Global Gag Rule', 1 February 2017, retrieved 19 June 2021 from https://www.awid.org/news-and-analysis/feminist-standpoints-global-gag-rule.
5. PAHO, 'Questions and Answers: Zika and Pregnancy', retrieve 19 June 2021 from https://www.paho.org/hq/index.php?option=com_content&view=article&id=11552:questions-and-answers-zika-and-pregnancy&Itemid=41711&lang=en.
6. LifeSiteNews, retrieved 19 June 2021 from https://www.lifesitenews.com/news/who-claims-zika-crisis-reveals-extreme-consequence-of-developing-nations-pr.

References

Adams, P. 2016. 'From Uruguay, a Model for Making Abortion Safer', *The New York Times*, 28 June.

Aiken, Abigail R.A., James G. Scott, Rebecca Gomperts, James Trussell, Marc Worrell and Catherine E. Aiken. 2016. 'Requests for Abortion in Latin America Related to Concern about Zika Virus Exposure', *New England Journal of Medicine* 375(4): 396–98.

Ali, M., K. Miller and R.F. Gómez Ponce de Leon. 2017. 'Family Planning and Zika Virus: Need for Renewed and Cohesive Efforts to Ensure Availability of Intrauterine Contraception in Latin America and the Caribbean', *The European Journal of Contraception & Reproductive Health Care* 22(2): 102–6.

Ali, S., et al. 2017. 'Environmental and Social Change Drive the Explosive Emergence of Zika Virus in the Americas', *PLOS Neglected Tropical Diseases* 11(2): e0005135.

Boseley, S. 2016. 'Zika Emergency Pushes Women to Challenge Brazil's Abortion Law', *The Guardian*, 19 July.

Camargo, T. 2016. 'The Debate on Abortion and Zika: Lessons from the AIDS Epidemic', *Cadernos de Saúde Pública* 32(5).

Carabali, M., et al. 2018. 'The Zika Epidemic and Abortion in Latin America: A Scoping Review', *Global Health Research and Policy* 3(1): 15.

CitizenGO. 2016. 'Don't Use the #Zika Virus to Push an Abortion Agenda!' Retrieved 27 February 2021 from http://www.citizengo.org/en/lf/32813-dont-use-zika-virus-push-abortion-agenda.

De Campos, T.C. 2016. 'Zika, Public Health, and the Distraction of Abortion', *Medicine, Health Care and Philosophy* 20(3): 443–46.

Diniz, D. 2016a. 'The Zika Virus and Brazilian Women's Right to Choose', *The New York Times*, 8 February.

——. 2016b. 'Zika Virus and Women', *Cadernos de Saúde Pública* 32(5): e00046316. Epub 13 May.

Diniz, D., et al. 2017. 'Zika Virus Infection in Brazil and Human Rights Obligations', *International Journal of Gynecology & Obstetrics* 136(1): 105–10.

Fegan, E.V., and R. Rebouche. 2003. 'Northern Ireland's Abortion Law: The Morality of Silence and the Censure of Agency', *Feminist Legal Studies* 11(3): 221–54.

Fernandes Moron, A. 2017. 'Zika Virus Outbreak and Reproductive Rights', *BJOG: An International Journal of Obstetrics & Gynaecology* 124(4): 549.

Garcia Jones, G. 2016. 'False Alarm over Zika Virus Leads to Untold Unnecessary Abortions', *LifeSite News*, 1 November.

Goldthwaite, L.M., and G. Velasquez. 2016. 'Family Planning and the Zika Era', *Current Opinion in Obstetrics and Gynecology* 28(6): 499–503.

González Vélez, A.C., and S.G. Diniz. 2016. 'Inequality, Zika Epidemics, and the Lack of Reproductive Rights in Latin America', *Reproductive Health Matters* 24(48): 57–61.

Gruskin, S., D. Bogecho and L. Ferguson. 2010. '"Rights-Based Approaches" to Health Policies and Programs: Articulations, Ambiguities, and Assessment', *Journal of Public Health Policy* 31(2): 129–45.

Heymann, D., et al. 2016. 'Zika Virus and Microcephaly: Why Is This Situation a PHEIC?', *The Lancet* 387(10020): 719–21.

Hodge, J.G., Jr. 2016. 'Generation Zika', *Jurimetrics* 57: 25–43.

Huetteman, E., and S. Tavernise. 2016. 'Senate Democrats Block Zika Bill over Planned Parenthood Provisions', *The New York Times*, 7 September.

Krisch, Joshua A. 2016. 'When a Country without Abortion Tells Women Not to Get Pregnant', Vocativ, 25 January. Retrieved 18 June 2021 from http://www.vocativ.com/275592/el-salvador-pregnancy-ban/.

Kumar, A., L. Hessini and E. Mitchell. 2009. 'Conceptualising Abortion Stigma', *Culture, Health & Sexuality* 11(6): 625–39.

Langer, A., J.M. Caglia and C. Menéndez. 2016. 'Sexual and Reproductive Health and Rights in the Time of Zika in Latin America and the Caribbean', *Studies in Family Planning* 47(2): 179–81.

Leite, M. 2016. 'The Outbreak of the Zika Virus and Reproductive Rights in Latin America', *E-International Relations*, 24 February.

McNeil, D.G., Jr. 2016. 'WHO Clarifies Advice on Sex and Pregnancy in Zika Regions', *The New York Times*, 7 September.

———. 2017. 'How the Response to Zika Failed Millions', *The New York Times*, 16 January.
McNeil, Donald G., Jr. and Julia Symmes Cobb. 2016. 'Colombia Is Hit Hard by Zika, But Not by Microcephaly', *The New York Times*, 31 October.
Meier, B.M., and A.S. Ayala. 2014. 'The Pan American Health Organization and the Mainstreaming of Human Rights in Regional Health Governance', *The Journal of Law, Medicine & Ethics* 42(3): 356–74.
Morgan, L.M., and E.F.S. Roberts. 2012. 'Reproductive Governance in Latin America', *Anthropology & Medicine* 19(2): 241–54.
Phillips, D., and N. Miroff. 2016. 'Scientists Are Bewildered by Zika's Path across Latin America', *The Washington Post*, 25 October.
Roa, M. 2016. 'Zika Virus Outbreak: Reproductive Health and Rights in Latin America', *The Lancet* 387: 843.
Román, V. 2016. 'Zika Awakens Debate over Legal and Safe Abortion in Latin America', *Scientific American*, 23 February.
Singh, J.A., and S.S. Abdool Karim. 2017. 'Trump's "Global Gag Rule" Implications for Human Rights and Global Health', *The Lancet* 5(4): 387–89.

Chapter 10
Figures of Drug-Resistant Tuberculosis

Jens Seeberg, Bijayalaxmi Rautaray and Shyama Mohapatra

It is possible to understand antimicrobial resistance (AMR) as an undesired product of over- and underuse of antibiotics in much the same way as, for example, air pollution is a product of diesel- and petrol-driven car transportation, landslides are products of deforestation on mountain slopes, and hormonal abnormalities are products of phthalates used in plastics and cosmetics. AMR, then, is a product of particular patterns of interaction between microbes, medicines and humans. From such a perspective, the concept of configuration points to a distributed production facility alongside the positive effects of antimicrobial use, allowing AMR production to take place on a large scale. Analysing antimicrobial resistance as a configuration from this angle would, we suggest, entail studying the product, its production and (importantly) its reproduction in a reinforcing feedback process in which resistance is simultaneously configured and configuring.

We build our argument on Jens Seeberg's work among private and public healthcare providers in Odisha in 2004–09 and as a researcher within the TB control programme in 2003–05. More recently, over a period of eighteen months in 2015–18, we collaborated in multisited fieldwork in which we engaged with twenty patients with drug-resistant tuberculosis. We visited them regularly during short-term fieldwork, we witnessed their suffering (and in some cases their recovery), and we learned from their narratives about their life circumstances, their providers and the development of their disease. In this chapter, we think about their lives through the idea of configuration in continuation of discussions at the Aarhus Center for Cultural Epidemics (EPICENTER) that lead Jens Seeberg to suggest that AMR transgresses the biomedical distinction between communicable and non-communicable diseases and this is also true for drug-resistant tuberculosis (DRTB). We argue that it is too simple to see the mutation in a bacterial cell that establishes resistance to a particular drug as the 'ultimate origin' of drug resistance. Instead, we should focus more on the configurations that enable this transmutation. Without the primary role of such configurations, AMR would be nothing but a relatively rare event and not the fast-growing public health crisis that we witness, even if it is briefly overshadowed by the coronavirus pandemic – an issue that we shall return to in the final section.

Context and Configuring

'Context is and always has been the key anthropological concept', asserted Ladislav Holy (1999: 48), and he proceeded to discuss contextualization as a necessary component, a sine qua non, of interpretation and, by the same token, a result of that interpretation. Citing Hobart, context can be seen as an analytical convenience designed for a particular purpose. In the same volume, entitled *The Problem of Context*, Dilley discussed Derrida's position that 'no meaning can be determined out of context, but no context permits saturation', as well as Culler's comment on this: 'meaning is context-bound but context is boundless' (Dilley 1999: 22). In many ways, the centrality of this foundational problem is what makes anthropology both tremendously rich in its contributions to understanding the world, and at times frustratingly open-ended in this potentially utopian task.

One may see the concept of configuring as an analytical handle to address Dilley's problem of context – not in any dogmatic sense, but as a tool that can inform the direction in which one looks when deciding on the relevance of context. Beyond what Hobart called 'analytical convenience', configuration can dissolve this distinction between a text and its potentially never-ending but meaning-generating context, and instead try to understand the circumstances, structures, elements and actions that combine into necessary preconditions for resistance to develop – not in any unidirectional causality, but in a relational web that we call configuration. Rather than figure and ground, we think of configuring processes as multitudes of interacting figures, akin to assemblage in DeLanda's 'assemblage theory 2.0' (DeLanda 2006), and maintaining a similarly realist stance but perhaps giving more emphasis to the human level of ontology, since, after all, we are still around.

As suggested in the introduction to this volume, we borrow the term 'configuration' from Rosenberg (1992), who has proposed it as one of several terms (together with contagion and contamination) to describe epidemics. He used the term in two slightly different ways. One is configuration as a type of pre-biomedical explanatory model: 'Before physicians had any knowledge of specific infectious agents, medical explanations of epidemic disease tended to be holistic and inclusive: an epidemic was the consequence of a unique configuration of circumstances, a disturbance in a 'normal' – health-maintaining and health-constituting – arrangement of climate, environment, and communal life' (Rosenberg 1992: 295). While anthropology may have partially renounced the ambition of holism, we can perhaps pursue the idea of the configuration of circumstances. Rather than being 'unique' (Rosenberg's term), a configuration may be *particular*, as in his example of Florence Nightingale, in which he states: 'She endorsed the traditional and seemingly common-sense notion that a sufficiently intense level of atmospheric contamination could induce both endemic and epidemic ills in the hospital's crowded wards (with particular configurations of environmental circumstance determining which)' (Rosenberg 1992: 96). In this Nightingale example, a configurationist explanation is not an alternative to contamination as in the previous quote. Instead, configurations explain the circumstances in which contamination happens. However, in a brief discussion of typhus as understood in the mid-nineteenth century, Rosenberg points to the contemporary use of the notion of 'contingent contagion' to describe 'the aggregate of local circumstances ... [that] interacted to create a particularly malignant microenvironment, one that detracted from the vitality of individuals and concentrated the increasingly disordered organic exudates from both sick and well' (Rosenberg 1992: 298). We suggest that this pre-biomedical notion of contingent contagion may be helpful in terms of rethinking the spread of AMR as happening in configurations that must be understood to include *both* the specifics of the epidemic that we seek to understand, including biosocial dynamics linking the cell, the body and human sociality, *and* what Rosenberg calls environment in the Nightingale example – which we would tend to see as structural figures that join to form a historically particular configuration of tuberculosis.

Tuberculosis

Tuberculosis (TB) is curable with antibiotic treatment. In spite of this fact, it currently has the highest mortality among infectious diseases globally.[1] In 2014, the World Health Organization (WHO) launched a new TB control strategy known as the 'End TB Strategy', aiming to reduce TB deaths by 95 per cent and to cut new cases by 90 per cent between 2016 and 2035, and, as they boldly state, 'to ensure that no family is burdened with catastrophic expenses due to TB'.[2] These agreeable but optimistic goals depend both on new technological developments in TB diagnosis, prevention and treatment, and on universal access to effective healthcare services incorporating these improvements. But as we shall see, standard public health approaches do not seem to be adequate if the goals of the WHO are to be met successfully.

One-third of the world's 7.5 billion people (2.5 billion people) are already infected with TB, and 5–10 per cent of them will develop active TB at some point. This corresponds to 125–250 million people, if no further transmission were to occur, so the new TB control strategy is attempting to address a formidable challenge. New strains of DRTB have emerged, and the spread of DRTB is rapidly becoming a global crisis, effectively cancelling out the reductions in prevalence that had otherwise been achieved in TB control, even though the introduction of repurposed and new drugs such as Bedaquiline has improved the chance of survival for DRTB patients.

DRTB may be treatment-generated (i.e. caused by the treatment given to the individual patient) or transmission-generated (spreading in a population). Correct diagnosis both in terms of whether or not a patient is suffering from TB and whether or not positive cases are infected with a drug-susceptible or drug-resistant strain remains a problem in spite of recent technological advances. This continues to be a substantial problem in India, which is home to a quarter of the global TB burden, not least because of the dominant influence of private actors involved in various ways in healthcare service of dubious quality (Seeberg 2012, 2013).

In the remaining part of this chapter, we shall explore the dynamics of contingent contagion as it configures drug-resistant tuberculosis in the state of Odisha, India. This configuring involves different actors, including bacteria, drugs, patients, families, providers and programme managers. We propose a set of four figures that interact to produce DRTB, namely pharmakon, regimen, klinikē and oikonomia, but space allows only for discussion of the first two in some detail.

Pharmakon

In Derrida's analysis of Plato's *Phaedrus*, where Socrates is led astray by Phaedrus' promise of 'volumes of speeches', what is at stake is the primacy of the spoken word in comparison to the epiphenomenon of writing (Derrida 1981). During the interaction, Socrates tells a story about the invention of writing in ancient Egypt. In brief, the story goes, the Egyptian Moon God, Thoth, offers to King Thamus the gift of writing, claiming his 'invention is a recipe (pharmakon) for both memory and wisdom'. But the king, whose spoken word is law, for which reason he has no need of writing, rejects the present, saying, 'The fact is that this invention will produce forgetfulness in the souls of those who have learned it because they will not need to exercise their memories. ... So it's not a remedy for memory, but for reminding, that you have discovered. And as for wisdom, you're equipping your pupils with only a semblance of it, not with truth' (Derrida 1981: 102). *Writing* is a pharmakon, an ambiguous drug, constituting its opposite, salvaging the life of the spoken word by 'putting it to sleep in a monument', presumably referring to a sarcophagus and the association of Thoth with death. The recipe, the writing, the pharmakon constitutes both a remedy and a poison at the same time.

With this in mind, let me briefly turn to the field of microbiological inscriptions. A virus is a string of DNA, a bit of genetic code if not text, in search of a cellular page on which it can write itself. Phages are such viruses that look for 'bacterial books', and mycobacterial phages search for TB to be rewritten. The phage is itself a naturally occurring microbiological pharmakon. From the perspective of Mycobacterium tuberculosis, anti-tuberculosis drugs have certain similarities to phages, but they are also dissimilar in important ways. Drugs are not viral, they do not replicate, and so the person under treatment must consume them for a long period. Nevertheless, medicines can be considered similar to phages in terms of the natural response of the cell to develop mechanisms that enable it to resist the specific mode of operation of a given drug (Seeberg 2020a). And, like Derrida's pharmakon, they may be a remedy or a poison from the bacterial perspective: if the treatment is effective, they become a poison to the bacteria. However, under certain circumstances they become a remedy against further treatment, as the bacteria may develop drug resistance. Once resistance is developed, the genetic material of the TB cell has changed, and subsequently this degree of drug resistance is replicated through standard processes of cell division. In other words, the pharmakon has the capacity to write into the bacteria the remedy against itself. This allows for new resistant strains of TB to spread both within the human host and, if it is infectious pulmonary TB, to other hosts.

In the case of the pharmakon of the standard TB regimen, the lives of two organisms are at stake: the lives of the Mycobacterium tuberculosis bacilli, and the life of their host. Both are simultaneously contaminated by the toxic treatment. The use of combination treatment in this regimen is intended to kill the bacteria and prevent drug resistance more effectively, but their combined toxicity also frequently results in side effects for the patient, including head reeling, vomiting, itching, rashes, weakness, and discolouration of urine. Sometimes, some of these side effects disappear over time, perhaps as an expression of bodily resistance to the toxins. But the disciplining of the regimen and the paternalism of the supervision are hard to live through for some. We have followed twenty patients with DRTB, which hardly constitutes a strong statistical foundation; but it is striking that when we met them more than half of them were below twenty-seven years of age, the youngest being eighteen, perhaps indicating a higher risk of development of drug resistance among younger TB patients. For this age group their difficulties in subjecting themselves to the regimen were intertwined with the increasing will to make independent decisions in early adulthood, a life stage during which decisions to move for the sake of work, education or the excitement of independent life easily generate resistance to the paternalism of supervised treatment during the intensive phase of treatment. The story of Batuk illustrates this. He was nineteen and in tenth grade when diagnosed with TB. Living in poverty in a *'basti'* (slum settlement) in a large city, he was the best-educated member of his family and considered the brightest of three brothers. His DOT provider ('DOTS' being the strategy recommended by the WHO for the control of TB, and standing for 'directly observed treatment, short-course') was a relative who delivered the medicines and left without checking if he actually took them. At first Batuk took these medicines, but (as he later explained) he had not been informed of the implications of interrupted treatment and so he stopped taking the medicine when he began to feel better to concentrate on his plans to get married. It was a love marriage, and he went ahead despite the disapproval of his mother. Around four months had passed without medicine when he started coughing blood. When he went to hospital, he was severely reprimanded and labelled as a 'defaulter'. The term is normally applied to someone who does not pay his bills and hence is unreliable and not to be trusted in the future. But in TB treatment the label was used for someone who had failed to observe a treatment regimen and was therefore associated with the same negative qualities as the bad payer. At this point Batuk was diagnosed with DRTB, and the doctor made sure to write 'chronic defaulter' on his file.

The concept of pharmakon captures the ambivalence of the toxic treatment with pathological effects for either human host or disease. In his analysis of the practice of 'Mohit', a practitioner of medicine without formal medical qualifications, McDowell uses Derrida's concept of pharmakon to understand the widespread symptomatic treatment in India. He suggests that this practitioner's 'pharmakon questions unidirectional relationships between knowing and treating disease or symptom. Examining connections between pharmaceuticals, symptom, disease, and knowledge suggests Mohit and many others' practice is a pharmakon that heals and endangers, knows and distorts the body and illness, and fosters and imperils life' (McDowell 2017: 335). General expectations that medicines should relieve rather than cause suffering may play a role in TB treatment. However, in the case of TB – and DRTB in particular – the detailed regulation and control of the composition of the pharmakon is vital. We discuss this dimension of the configuration of DRTB through the figure of 'regimen'.

Regimen

Regimen, from Latin *regere*, 'to rule', and in late Middle English denoting the action of governing, means 'a prescribed course of medical treatment, diet, or exercise for the promotion or restoration of health', according to the Oxford Dictionary of English.[3] For many years, the regimen of standard TB medicines, known as DOTS, has consisted of four TB drugs. India has recently switched officially to a daily regimen, but during most of the period of data collection on which this article is based, DOTS was given every second day. Missing one dose meant missing three days of treatment, which could increase the risk of treatment-generated drug resistance. To prevent this risk, treatment is subject to direct observation provided by a so-called DOT provider.

While some find the TB regimen difficult to adhere to, the challenge of subjecting oneself to the DRTB regimen is much greater. Consisting of six drugs in the intensive phase of six to nine months, and four drugs in the continuation phase of eighteen months, and involving significant risks of liver and kidney damage and permanent hearing impairment, this regimen comes with serious side effects. These can be compared with the side effects of oncological chemotherapy, except that the drugs used to treat DRTB are administered daily, for two years, and by the patients themselves, who (apart from an injection that has to be given at the health centre) often collect medicines for a week at a time and divide the day into sleep, medicine intake and vomiting. In addition, a number of medicines are prescribed to address some of the toxic effects of the pharmakon, such as anti-acidics and Ayurvedic liver tonics, not to mention the ever-present cough syrup.

Diya was in her early twenties and diagnosed with DRTB. Diya's brother Subrat was seventeen years old and was earning his contribution to the household economy as an assistant in a medicine store when he started coughing badly in December 2013. Not surprisingly in his trade, he started taking medicines that were readily available from the shop, and his employer, the owner of the store, also helped identify combinations of drugs that could cover anything from the common cold and upper respiratory infections to asthma. But his cough continued, and after two to three months of ineffective treatment he went to the private clinic of Jeroo Madam, one of the senior doctors in the pulmonary medicine department of a large government hospital in Odisha. Dr Jeroo did not initiate standard diagnostic procedures at the government hospital, where she worked during the day, but sent him to a private clinic for an X-ray, blood tests and a sputum test costing Rs. 2,500, or €35. A TB diagnosis was confirmed, and Subrat started the expensive treatment through Dr Jeroo's private clinic even though she could have chosen to give Subrat the medicine for free from the government hospital. This would have been an advantage for Subrat, who also lost his job at the medicine store due to his condition. However, Dr Jeroo did not prescribe the standard regimen recommended by the WHO, which consisted of four drugs and was considered difficult to take by some patients due to side effects. Instead, she prescribed a combination tablet widely available in India under the name AKT2. This pharmakon is less toxic and easier to consume than the standard regimen, but the risk of treatment-generated drug resistance is considerably higher because AKT2 only contains two active components instead of the recommended four components, and a few months later Subrat was diagnosed with DRTB.

Around this time, Subrat's sister Diya started coughing badly. She also went to Dr Jeroo, who sent her to the same private facilities for TB testing, and she, too, was found to be TB-positive. She was given the same TB treatment that had not cured her brother. When we first met her, she was coughing frequently even though she had been under treatment for several months and had paid tens of thousands of Rupees for this treatment, which was supposed to be free. She had believed Dr Jeroo's assurance that 'if you will buy the medicine from "outside", it will be much better than the government one'. We advised her to be tested for DRTB.

When we met three months later, she recounted what had happened. Originally, when she had seen Dr Jeroo, who knew that her brother had DRTB, the doctor had told her, 'It's normal TB, you don't need to worry'.[4] When she returned and asked for a DRTB test, the doctor said, 'Oh sorry, I forgot [that your brother has

DRTB]'. Feeling that the doctor had betrayed her trust, she decided to change to another doctor at the government hospital. Her TB also proved to be drug resistant and had probably been transmitted from her brother. During subsequent interviews, Diya took care to wear a mask. Unfortunately, Dr Jeroo had not advised her brother to do the same when he was diagnosed with drug-resistant TB.

While Dr Jeroo may have felt she was simply taking care of her private business, she also seemed to demonstrate a strong preference for a costly but ineffective regimen at very high financial and health cost to patients like Diya and Subrat. If Subrat had been treated effectively, he and his sister might not have developed DRTB at all. When Diya belatedly started the DRTB treatment, she described in her diary how she felt her life was gradually being poisoned.

> 24 May 2016. Then while starting to have the medicines I vomited; then sometime after having the medicines I vomited; and like this till night I vomited and due to this the taste of my mouth changed. I only had the bitter taste in my mouth. I felt like my head was spinning, then weakness, then the pain in my body was so much that I was not able to walk on my own. I got so irritated that I didn't want to listen to or see to anything. Everything feels like poison. I didn't wish to eat but I had to because after my food I had to take the medicine. Then I took it. Then now I am trying to sleep but sleep is not coming. Weird thoughts are coming to my mind.

Later on, she said that people from whom she had expected care spoke to her in 'a hateful tone', so that 'every happiness of the world becomes poison'. 'To cure someone's pain, medicines are blessings', she wrote, 'but ... this medicine is poison for the patients'. For Diya, the combination of the unbearable side effects – these are only described briefly here – and the lack of social support from her boyfriend, whom she eventually left, and from her mother and two siblings, to whose house she had returned during the course of treatment, combined to poison not only her body but her entire life as a social being, and she became increasingly depressed and suicidal. Eventually she decided to stop her treatment as a way out of this situation, getting back to a life in which she could be active, earn a living, and have the courage to end a relationship with a violent boyfriend whose nightly stone-throwing caused her family to relocate. She felt that she was embracing life again, but she also knew that not taking the medicine was potentially a slow form of suicide – if the disease returned. Whereas the drug resistance of her disease had been addressed through a toxic contamination of her body and of her life, her own resistance to the medicines was a bodily and social detoxification project based on yoga and Ayurvedic treatment, and breaking the social isolation that she suffered during treatment. It was also an active rejection of the medical system – which she perceived as systematically exploitative and faulty: irregular drug supply, the provision of bad drugs, and rude and unsupportive behaviour that created additional barriers for her access to the medicines, all formed part of the configuration of her DRTB. When we last met her, she looked healthy and happy, but we both knew that the possibility of relapse could not be ruled out.

In Diya's case, resistance was a strategy of short-term survival and making life not only bearable but worth living again. Let me now return to Batuk, whose DRTB was probably caused by irregular treatment at the age of nineteen, at a point in time when he was preoccupied with marriage and the related family conflict. At age twenty-two, when we first met him, he was struggling with the side effects of the medicines and with the ill health of their infant daughter. He lived with his wife and daughter in a one-room house adjacent to the tiny houses of his brother and his parents in a *basti* in a large city, squeezed between a rubbish dump, a drain and a cowshed. Reading Batuk's diary provides insight into a life punctuated by an almost churning monotony of waking up, having some of the little food that may be available, having medicines, vomiting, feeling unwell, sleeping, waking up, going to a health post for injections, returning unwell, quarrelling with family members because of his inability to work, somebody needing money, nobody having any, playing with his daughter, worrying for her. But occasionally, and no matter how ill he was, Batuk took any other sick family member to the hospital or picked up medicine for them from the chemist. His disease had turned him into a local expert in health system interaction. And a critical expert, as he was keenly aware of the catastrophic costs his disease had inflicted on the household, and equally critical of the extraction of money from poor patients that he witnessed for himself and for others – despite the fact that all medicines and tests were supposed to be free for DRTB patients. In his words:

> Going to the big hospital [the doctor] is writing for injection for [INR] 500, 1,000 [EUR 6.5; 13] one, one injection… for one needle. That syringe, for 8–10 days that you have to stay. Before it was free, now they are saying 'for as many days you are staying here, buy the syringe'… 'buy the needle' … Everything was free in 2013 and 2014, but now in 2015 they are telling [me] to buy everything… if we are not buying then they make us leave… for all reports it's [INR] 500, 1,000, 1,500, 2,000, 5,000. Like this they are saying.

While there may be a need to send patients to private clinics which are located conveniently near the hospital for additional tests that are not available at the government hospital, poor patients like Batuk are entitled to reimbursement. Like other patients we met who had filed claims and submitted their bills, he had received no reimbursement. Often bills got 'lost' in the process.

Extracting money from DRTB patients was part of the configuration of the DRTB epidemic and had the effect of co-constructing the regimen in ways that undermined successful treatment for poor patients like Batuk by limiting access to a healthy diet required to compensate for weight loss; to medicines, especially ancillary drugs for side effects; and to tests essential to the ongoing monitoring and adjustment of medication. For example, Batuk described his inability to get routine X-ray and blood test examinations:

> They [the doctors] have told me to do the test [X-ray and various blood tests] for around INR 2,000 [USD32]. It's now three days. I don't have money, so I am not doing that. Let's see what will I do, they have written… all my chest is paining, means heart… heart problem is there so that's why I cannot control… sometimes I couldn't breathe, I just sit in the bed like this for half an hour… one hour… feeling weak… then also when I cough my heart aches… … I really don't have money so I didn't do it… they told to come within one hour but now it's three days… they are calling but what can I do, I don't have money… if money would have been there, then I would have done it… I don't have money even to have medicine.

Some months later, Batuk collapsed. Unable to breathe, he was admitted to the DRTB ward. His brother sold the little dowry gold the family possessed to fund an admission process that was supposed to be free of charge under government regulations. After one month, Batuk had regained enough strength to return home, but he was still feverish and extremely weak. He was coughing constantly, and a culture test showed that his disease had evolved into extensively drug-resistant TB known as XDRTB, a condition that had a very poor prognosis in spite of an extremely toxic regimen with dramatic side effects. Despite his poor health, he monitored the treatment he was given critically and lamented the absence of the pulmonologists at the ward, where people were examined only by medical students. An expert patient, he was able to describe the errors that occurred and the resulting treatment irregularities precisely:

> I have started taking Capreomycin[5] [for XDRTB] for the last three months. ... There are four months left. I am taking the medicines, but they are being careless, I mean, the person who is giving medicines... I have [to take] only ten tablets. At times, they give ten tablets and at other times eight. It depends on their mood. I complained about it. There, I said, 'Sir! Why are you giving me medicines in this manner? You can see that I am a patient. I am continuing the medicines. Why don't you give me medicine?' They say, 'We don't remember. We give these medicines. Now, you take them. We will give you [the rest] later'. What does this mean? I'll have eight tablets but, not the complete course. Which also means that I'll take half of them. Ultimately, it will make me ill, for which reason my health is deteriorating. So, what is the use of having so many medicines? I complained about those two medicines one month ago. ... Till now, they are not giving. They are only providing eight medicines. When I complain, they never listen.

Even so, someone must have noticed that the regimen was not being fully implemented, and a delegation consisting of a doctor, supervisor and his DOT provider visited his house and blamed him for his erroneous regimen.

> They are asking me to show what kind of medicines I am taking; and in turn they are scolding me a lot. When I am explaining the things that have taken place, they are still blaming me. They are also telling me, 'Who told you to decrease the quantity of the medicines? Why do you decrease the quantity at your own will?' ... At times, they are giving large tablets and at other times small ones. Can't I recognize the tablet that I am taking regularly? If I complain to them about it, they are saying, 'What do you know? We are always giving you the same tablets'. Then, I told [the doctor], 'You are giving me the tablets. It's fine. But, you are not giving it with your own hands; you have a person for that. That person is giving me the tablets and I am taking them. You are seeing my face once in a week. ... But, I am seeing this every time. Can't I recognize my medicines?' ... They are reducing the amount of medicines.

Figures of Drug-Resistant Tuberculosis

Batuk knew that if he died the family would have no resources to support his wife and small daughter, who meant everything to him. Again and again, he repeated that he was taking the medicines for the sake of his daughter, and that he was putting up with the side effects for her. What he could not tolerate was the thought that he would die because of the carelessness of the service providers who were in charge of the administration of the XDRTB regimen, and he found ways to take the medicines himself directly from the storeroom at the health centre. He had also built up a reserve stock at his house, enough to keep him going for five days in case stocks of his drugs ran out at the health centre. His resistance was not to the medicine, but to the faults in the system. Even so, he was still labelled as a defaulter in his hospital reports, as a warning that he was not a patient to be trusted.

Configuration of Drug-Resistant Tuberculosis in India

Drug resistance transgresses the distinction between communicable and non-communicable disease (Seeberg and Meinert 2015). Drug resistance as a biological phenomenon can be regarded as a process of contamination – bacteria mutating in response to exposure to toxic substances – or as contagion, because if the treatment has no effect, these same bacteria can be infectious. However, the categories of treatment-generated and transmission-generated DRTB are not mutually exclusive,[6] and the configuration of production of drug resistance mirrors their interlinked complexities. In this chapter, we have looked at specific figures that co-produce this configuration on the basis of a central premise: at the centre of the configuration is the patient who is subjected to the workings of the figures, as these interact in the situated local biologies (Niewöhner and Lock 2018) of both patients and the TB bacteria they harbour.

From the stories of Diya and Batuk, dynamic figures of biosocial resistance that co-produce the configuration of DRTB across species, substances and social categories begin to emerge in a context of immediate biopolitical and socioeconomic environments as well as global TB control policies. We shall end by briefly summarizing four figures of the configuration: pharmakon, regimen, regula, klinikē and oikonomia.

As should be clear from the above, *pharmakon* in the context of TB points to the balancing of cross-species toxicity for bacteria and human host. This balance determines the difference between cure and death for both, favouring only one or the other. The pharmakon's balance changes over time, with successful treatment of susceptible TB favouring the human host, and increasing levels of drug resistance favouring the bacteria and at the same time increasing the stakes as the pharmakon's toxicity increases, creating increasingly debilitating side effects for the patient. As Diya told us, and as revealed by the narratives of most DRTB patients we have met, the poison often spilled over and coloured the mind, which became depressive and resigned to fate (see also Seeberg 2020b). But social relations were also poisoned by the combined impact of disease and treatment. When an XDRTB patient dies, it may not be clear whether the direct cause of death should be attributed to TB, to the pharmakon or to their combined impact.

The *regimen* for drug-susceptible TB is designed to ensure that the balance of the pharmakon tips in favour of the human host of TB disease. With increasing resistance levels, including microbacterial, social and economic resistances, this goal becomes increasingly difficult and sometimes desperate. The regimen implies *regula*, rules, as well as implying specific forms of adherence that distinguish compliant patients from defaulters, that is, rule breakers who, once labelled, are seen as less deserving and unlikely to be cured by the pharmakon and therefore can be given less attention. While such stigmatizing processes are at odds with global TB control recommendations and guidelines, they can be difficult to eradicate because they merge with a host of other social dynamics influencing the way in which a patient is treated, including caste, gender, income and educational factors. But from a different perspective, regula also implies policy implementation, including the provision of free treatment and diagnostics and the reimbursement of medical expenses when free services are not accessible. Non-compliance among health providers, combined with the fact that some doctors practise in both the public and private sectors, blurs the distinction between these two sectors and points to the figure of *klinikē*, the clinic (from Greek klinikē (tekhnē), 'bedside (art)', from klinē, 'bed') as the site of medical care. Government facilities are widely used to recruit customers – no matter how desperate and poor they are – to the largely unregulated private sector. This sector remains a key contributor to the production of drug resistance through non-standard treatment practices that are believed to increase the chances of retaining patients as customers. This feat requires careful consideration of costs and side effects, until, if DRTB develops, patients are handed over to the government facilities because they become too risky to have as private patients, or because the treatment becomes too expensive and/or unavailable in the private market. Lastly, the figure of *oikonomia* (household management, from oikos, 'house') incorporates the household as the site of financial, emotional, social and intellectual resources. For many, in spite of policies establishing free treatment, TB involves a dramatic depletion of financial resources due to the insatiable demands of the clinic, draining the ability of poor households to manage basic food needs, a vital influence on the toxic balance of the *pharmakon*. The depletion of household finances and increasing levels of drug resistance in TB help to generate a syndemic of DRTB and social isolation, depression and suicide risk.

However, as Butler reminds us, resistance is not the opposite of vulnerability (Butler 2016). On the contrary, she says, vulnerability may be what brings about resistance, at least when we are talking about resistance as political mobilization. Butler makes it clear that she is not speaking about disease, even though she agrees that the consistent failure of infrastructures increases vulnerability. The mutuality of resistance and vulnerability is precarious under the figures outlined above: being infected with DRTB means finding yourself in a situation of extreme vulnerability. But as Diya and Batuk have shown, resistance can be an important part of that vulnerability. Their actions of opposition and rejection also partially shape the configuration of the epidemic of drug-resistant TB in this locality. Rather than demonstrating the vulnerability in resistance, these actions force us to inverse the focus due to the extreme precariousness of their lives to be able to talk about resistance in vulnerability instead.

Postscript: COVID-19 Configuring DRTB

The distribution of vulnerabilities and resources to cope with a public health crisis like the coronavirus varied widely among and within countries prior to its outbreak, and the pandemic has only widened pre-existing inequities. However, the unexpected impact of coronavirus in the world's richest countries has resulted in unprecedented investments in vaccine development, with the first citizens being vaccinated in countries such as the USA and the UK in late 2020. In contrast, we may celebrate the 100-year anniversary for the first BCG vaccine against TB given to a human in 1921 (Brimnes 2016). In spite of its low efficacy at 50 per cent (Colditz et al. 1994), no new vaccine has been developed since. Furthermore, it is striking that pharmaceutical companies have developed no new first-line drugs for more than fifty years, even if the *annual* death toll of this disease in the global south almost matches that of Covid-19 and has done for decades. Might one hope that the new vaccine technologies developed for coronavirus may have spin-off effects in the form of novel vaccines for other diseases such as TB?

Meanwhile, the pandemic itself and the lockdown policies to control it reconfigured other diseases with epidemic potential. The WHO has reported a 25–30 per cent drop in TB case notification in India during 2020.[7] The complete lockdown of the country on 24 March 2020 initially seemed to slow the spread of the virus with testing capacity limited to urban centres. However, as millions of migrant workers had to leave the cities on overcrowded buses and trains or by foot in an attempt to reach their places of residence, the virus was effectively spread all over the sub-continent (Maji, Choudhari and Sushma 2020). The scenarios predicted in May 2020 by Manderson and Wahlberg (2020) pointing to the negative impact of isolation and lack of access to healthcare for people living with chronic conditions that was caused both by the pandemic and the policies to control it seem to have played out in ways that vary according to their particular configurations. As we write this section in early January 2021, it is still too early to assess how such scenarios have played out in India, so let us instead return to Batuk. We managed to get in touch with him in September 2020 via Zoom on a rather poor mobile connection. He was not well. He had completed his full course of Bedaquiline in April and was considered to be cured, but his haemoptysis resumed. In his own words, he vomited a bucket full of blood. With the help of the research team, he managed to be allowed to resume treatment on a different regimen.

Figures of Drug-Resistant Tuberculosis

When we talked with him, he was in his home. Batuk told us that he could barely walk due to breathlessness and pain, and because of the lockdown he had no money for food, travel or treatment. Three weeks later, in early October, he was admitted to hospital where he died, six years and six months after initiating TB treatment under the DOTS programme.

Jens Seeberg
Professor, Department of Anthropology
Aarhus University, Denmark

Bijayalaxmi Rautaray
Secretary cum Chief Executive
Sahayog, India

Shyama Mohapatra
Assistant Professor, Department of Anthropology
Model Degree College, Rayagada, Odisha, India

Notes

1. In 2020, TB may have been surpassed by COVID-19 in terms of mortality. According to the WHO, an estimated 1.4 million people died from TB in 2019 (https://www.who.int/news-room/fact-sheets/detail/tuberculosis#:~:text=Key%20facts,with%20tuberculosis(TB)%20worldwide, accessed on 5 January 2021) and approximately 1.8 million from COVID-19 (https://www.who.int/data/stories/the-true-death-toll-of-covid-19-estimating-global-excess-mortality, accessed on 21 June 2021) in 2020. However, actual figures are expected to be much higher. Due to syndemic interactions between the two, TB mortality may have increased in 2020.
2. WHO, 'End TB Strategy', http://www.who.int/tb/post2015_strategy/en/, accessed on 5 January 2021.
3. See https://en.oxforddictionaries.com/definition/regimen, accessed on 5 January 2021.
4. Drug-susceptible TB was generally described as 'normal TB', and drug-resistant TB as 'serious TB'.
5. Capreomycin is a second-line treatment used for active drug-resistant tuberculosis, given by injection.
6. The disease of a person originally infected with a drug-resistant strain of TB (transmission-generated) may develop additional forms of (treatment-generated) resistance.

7. WHO, 'Global TB Progress at Risk', 14 October 2020, https://www.who.int/news/item/14-10-2020-who-global-tb-progress-at-risk, accessed on 5 January 2021)

References

Brimnes, Niels. 2016. *Languished Hopes: Tuberculosis, the State, and International Assistance in Twentieth Century India*. Delhi: Orient Blackswan.

Butler, Judith. 2016. 'Rethinking Vulnerability and Resistance', in Judith Butler, Zeynep Gambetti and Leticia Sabsay (eds), *Vulnerability in Resistance*. Durham, NC: Duke University Press, pp. 12–27.

Colditz, Graham A., et al. 1994. 'Efficacy of BCG Vaccine in the Prevention of Tuberculosis: Meta-Analysis of the Published Literature', *JAMA* 271(9): 698–702. doi:10.1001/jama.1994.03510330076038.

DeLanda, Manuel. 2006. *A New Philosophy of Society: Assemblage Theory and Social Complexity*. New York: A&C Black.

Derrida, Jacques. 1981. *Dissemination*, trans. Barbara Johnson, vol. 331. Chicago: Chicago University Press.

Dilley, Roy. 1999. 'Introduction: The Problem of Context', in Roy Dilley (ed.), *The Problem of Context*. New York: Berghahn Books, pp. 1–46.

Holy, Ladislav. 1999. 'Contextualisation and Paradigm Shifts', in Roy Dilley (ed.), *The Problem of Context*. New York: Berghahn Books, pp. 47–60.

Maji, Avijit, Tushar Choudhari and M.B. Sushma. 2020. 'Implication of Repatriating Migrant Workers on COVID-19 Spread and Transportation Requirements', *Transportation Research Interdisciplinary Perspectives* 7: 100187. doi:https://doi.org/10.1016/j.trip.2020.100187.

Manderson, Lenore, and Ayo Wahlberg. 2020. 'Chronic Living in a Communicable World', *Medical Anthropology* 39(5): 428–39. doi:10.1080/01459740.2020.1761352.

McDowell, Andrew. 2017. 'Mohit's Pharmakon: Symptom, Rotational Bodies, and Pharmaceuticals in Rural Rajasthan', *Medical Anthropology Quarterly* 31(3): 332–48. doi:10.1111/maq.12345.

Niewöhner, Jörg, and Margaret Lock. 2018. 'Situating Local Biologies: Anthropological Perspectives on Environment/Human Entanglements', *BioSocieties* 13(4): 681–97.

Rosenberg, C.E. 1992. *Explaining Epidemics and Other Studies in the History of Medicine*. Cambridge: Cambridge University Press.

Seeberg, Jens. 2012. 'Connecting Pills and People: An Ethnography of the Pharmaceutical Nexus in Odisha, India', *Medical Anthropology Quarterly* 26(2): 182–200.

———. 2013. 'The Death of Shankar: Tuberculosis and Social Exclusion in a Poor Neighbourhood in Bhubaneswar, Odisha', in Kenneth Bo Nielsen, Marianne Fibiger Qvortrup and Uwe Skoda (eds), *Navigating Social Exclusion and Inclusion in Contemporary India and Beyond*. London: Anthem, pp. 207–26.

———. 2020a. 'Biosocial Dynamics of Multidrug-Resistant Tuberculosis: A Bacterial Perspective', in Jens Seeberg, Andreas Roepstorff and Lotte Meinert (eds), *Biosocial Worlds: Anthropology of Health Environments beyond Determinism*. London: UCL Press, pp. 124–45.

———. 2020b. 'Fear of Drug-Resistant Tuberculosis as Social Contagion', *Ethnos* 85(4): 665–78. doi:10.1080/00141844.2019.1634615.

Seeberg, Jens, and Lotte Meinert. 2015. 'Can Epidemics Be Non-Communicable? Reflections on the Spread of "Non-Communicable" Diseases', *Medicine Anthropology Theory* 2(2): 54–71.

Afterword
Epidemics and Ghosts
Byron J. Good

Introduction

This book is based on a provocative, even rather audacious claim: that when the term 'epidemic' is applied to noncommunicable diseases or conditions, such as obesity or suicide, it should be understood as a literal rather than metaphoric use of the term. The underlying argument running throughout the book is that it is critical to break down the neat distinctions between infectious and non-infectious diseases when analysing conditions that take on epidemic proportions, and that this has serious implications not only for investigations of so-called 'noncommunicable' diseases, NCDs, but for infectious or communicable diseases as well. This in turn calls into question what is meant by 'communicable'. This framing of 'epidemic' has important implications for the analysis of both infectious and non-infectious diseases. This book, made up of anthropological case studies, suggests a critical role for the place of ethnography in such studies of epidemics, a field often left almost exclusively to epidemiologists. Lying in the background, somewhat out of sight in this collection, is a fundamental critique of the dark history of classic public health models for responding to epidemics. This volume grows out of the work of Epicenter, the Centre for Cultural Epidemics, at Aarhus University, as a part of their larger programme of activities aimed at rethinking the meaning of 'epidemics'.

The structure of the book itself embodies this challenge to the neat distinction between communicable and noncommunicable diseases. While much of the book is devoted to what are classified as noncommunicable conditions – suicide, autism, obesity, trauma-related mental health problems, 'hysterical' spirit attacks, mental health problems associated with internet porn – the final two chapters analyse responses to the Zika virus infection and drug-resistant tuberculosis, suggesting that all of these share much in common and that there is value to analyses that cross this divide. The editors draw on the analytic categories proposed by historian Charles Rosenberg (1992) in his studies of epidemic diseases: 'configuration' theories common before the discovery of micro-organisms, and 'contagion' theories which have become dominant. They expand the notion 'contagion' to include, quite centrally, theories of 'social contagion', as well as the concept 'contamination', to broaden the concept of communicability beyond that of micro-organisms. And they explore making 'configuration' theories and analyses much more central to the understanding of both infectious and non-infectious diseases, communicable and noncommunicable conditions as classically understood. 'Configurational' analyses, sometimes drawing on the verbal term 'configuring' rather than the nominal term 'configuration' to focus attention on processes over structures, incorporate cultural, biosocial, biopolitical, policy and governmental processes to develop understandings of constellations of biosocial forces critical to understanding infectious disease epidemics as well as those of NCDs. These analyses are linked in the Introduction to the volume and in some chapters to the concept 'syndemics', syndromes of biosocial conditions that produce epidemics, proposed by Singer and Clair (2003). The editors challenged the authors of the chapters in this volume to think through their own work drawing on these concepts, expanding analyses of conditions that assume epidemic proportions, and developing terminologies and explanatory frames that break down the boundaries between 'real' or infectious disease epidemics and conditions that are described as epidemic in a 'metaphoric' sense.

It is important to acknowledge the timeliness of this collection of essays in the context of the global COVID-19 pandemic. The gathering from which the chapters in this volume originated was held in Aarhus in April 2017. Initial chapter drafts were written prior to the global spread of the current coronavirus. These analyses thus serve as a template for understanding the enormous variations in the pattern of the COVID pandemic and responses to it across nations, societies and social groups – policy responses, behavioural responses by members of particular social and political groups, specific structures associated, for example, with the care of elders or in indigenous communities, and the resulting configuration of morbidity and mortality associated with the pandemic. Complex analyses of these phenomena are underway. However, this pandemic makes starkly clear the importance of analyses of the most infectious of diseases and the forms that pandemics take in biosocial and configurational, as well as historical, terms. Only in this way can the enormous diversity of patterns of spread of the virus and the resulting rates of illness and death be understood.

This volume raises a number of critical questions that will frame my reflections in this Afterword. What is meant by 'biosocial configurations', and what is the value of, as well as limits to, understanding epidemics in these terms, whether they be infectious or non-infectious? Are there distinctive social constellations – or syndromes – that can be clearly identified, and what should be included within – or excluded from – such biosocial configurations? In what ways are these to be understood as causal, and how do analyses of such constellations contribute to public health, clinical care or policy interventions? What is meant by 'social contagion', as proposed in the Introduction? What might we mean by 'transmission' of non-infectious conditions, and how can this be demonstrated? What is the role of interpretive ethnographic research versus epidemiological research in the study of epidemics from the perspective proposed in this volume? And what do we make of recent claims that both epidemiological analyses and public health responses are deeply implicated in colonial histories? What do we make of the suggestion that epidemics are particular sites of haunting, as Cheryl Mattingly and her colleagues argue? In what way do ghosts of colonial and racialized pasts – and presents – make their appearance within policy responses, as well as local public responses, to threatening epidemics? In what ways are public health policies and epistemological constructs that support these policies based in colonial histories of public health and responding to epidemics? What are the relations among

Foucauldian biopolitical, post-colonial and hauntological analyses of epidemics, pandemics and responses to these? I will of course not attempt to answer these questions, but suggest that questions such as these need to be addressed with as much clarity as possible in order to move forward with the challenging analyses suggested by the Epicenter group and the chapters in this volume.

Epidemics, Biosocial Configurations, Contagion

World Mental Health: Problems and Priorities in Low-Income Countries (Desjarlais et al. 1995) is a book that grew out of an extended project led by Arthur Kleinman, surveying what was known about mental health problems in low resource settings and potential interventions, with the goal of increasing prioritization of mental health in funding and programme activities in global health. One of the conclusions of that report read as follows:

> ...*the problems reviewed singly in separate chapters are in fact most typically found in clusters of psychosocial problems.* Substance abuse, violence toward women and children, psychiatric sequelae such as depression, and health risks in adulthood for children so victimized are closely associated with one another. Community violence is linked to post-traumatic stress disorders, dislocation, and depression. These clusters need to be identified and investigated if we are to design effective strategies of prevention and treatment. (1995: 263–64; emphasis in original text)

As I read back over this conclusion, it reads as quite consonant with the overall efforts in this book to identify 'biosocial configurations' or constellations – here labelled 'clusters' – of interacting social and medical conditions that may be present in epidemic form under certain conditions. Many of the chapters fit rather closely with the goal of identifying and investigating such 'clusters', with a larger goal of designing strategies of prevention and treatment. For example, the two papers on the Acholi communities of Uganda, chapter 1 by Whyte and Oboke and chapter 6 by Williams and Meinert, demonstrate a specific constellation of factors that have led to distinctive patterns of suicide, particularly among men, and of domestic violence, alcoholism, and conflicts over land following the war between the Lord's Resistance Army and the Uganda army and the subsequent confinement of the Acholi people in IDP camps.

However, this volume and recent writing on epidemics suggest the limits to this formulation. In chapter 2, Lowe demonstrates the extreme local character of 'epidemic suicide' in Oceania, providing an important contrast to factors associated with suicide among Acholi. He recounts how expatriate analysts came to the conclusion that 'rapid social changes associated with political independence, economic development and increasing globalization placed many indigenous people in Oceania at risk for a host of mental and physical health problems'. Such an interpretation seems reasonable at first glance. However, Lowe suggests that these 'universalizing accounts' represent 'colonial and postcolonial anxieties about the ability of local, indigenous peoples to become independent modern societies in the western liberal style as opposed to recognizing the diverse modernities Oceanic peoples have already constructed for themselves'. He argues further that the meaning of 'self-harm' or suicide depends heavily upon locally constituted forms of the 'self', and that suicide attempts in Chuuk often represent efforts to negotiate crises in social relationships within which the self is embedded and mend damaged relations. The assertion of universalizing accounts thus represents knowledge-making that reproduces colonial and post-colonial relations of power, Lowe argues.

The call for identifying and investigating clusters of psychosocial processes in order to 'design effective strategies of prevention and treatment', as articulated in the world mental health report, suggests the potential for identifying 'configurations' with enough specificity to design interventions that go beyond the usual treatment of specific conditions such as depression or substance use and that might be extended beyond a single society to be an important goal of global mental health. This is one potential interpretation of the call for understanding epidemics of non-infectious conditions in terms of biosocial configurations. On the other hand, critiques of this approach, such as that outlined by Lowe, raise challenging questions about the potential for such projects to reproduce historical relations of coloniality. Lowe's argument links to recent critiques of global public health and epidemiological research as reproducing colonial forms of knowledge about containment and control of infectious conditions, an issue I will return to in the

Afterword

Conclusion of this Afterword. What then are the implications for investigating 'biosocial configurations' as called for by the editors of this volume? A review of the chapters points in important directions while raising further questions.

These chapters, grounded in ethnography, point to the importance of detailed local social and cultural shaping of configurations. The breakdown of patrilineal patrilocal marriage patterns among the Acholi in Uganda, particularly following the war and confinement in IDP camps, provides a compelling example of what might produce an epidemic of domestic violence, mental health problems and suicide. The chapter on Aceh by Grayman, Good and Good is a reminder that apparently Western terms such as 'trauma' may be imported and take on very critical local meanings. Grøn's analysis of family experiences of obesity in Denmark and the crucial role of *hygge*, a distinctive local cultural form of sociality, is a reminder that configurations associated with noncommunicable conditions need not occur only among the poor and marginalized, but may be associated with highly normative and valued patterns of social and affective interactions.

But these chapters all raise questions about what should be included within any particular configuration, whether only proximate and local processes should be included or whether more distal historical processes should be a part of all analyses. To what extent should British colonialism and the subsequent arms trade be included in the analysis of a suicide epidemic among Acholi men in Uganda? Jens Seeberg and colleagues (chapter 10) argue convincingly that antimicrobial resistance and the spread of drug-resistant tuberculosis is a product of interactions among microbes, medicines and humans, that the coexistence of a poorly funded public sector of clinical services and a private sector conspire to produce both 'overuse and underuse' of antibiotics and thus an epidemic of multi-drug-resistant TB. But if referrals from public services to physicians' own private clinics and the inability of patients to pay for the medications is a critical part of the configurations, are neoliberal economic policies, a vast discrepancy between rich and poor, and even colonial patterns of health services or the caste system a necessary part of such a configuration? Of course, at one level they are. But Seeberg and colleagues wisely quote an analysis of Derrida's arguments about meaning and context that 'meaning is context-bound but context is boundless' to make clear that what is included as belonging to a configuration depends on what the analysis of configuration is intended to speak to. Is this analysis essentially a piece of critical anthropology or comparative sociology, a contribution to advocacy for particular public health policies in India, or part of an effort to improve clinical practice?

Lynn Morgan (chapter 9) demonstrates that the pattern of Zika virus infection and the resulting levels of microcephaly in Brazil, particularly among the poorest women, cannot be understood without including the Pan American Health Organization's determination to 'avoid politics' associated with anti-abortion advocacy. Precisely by configuring the Zika epidemic in a narrowly conservative and technocratic manner, rather than serving as advocates for the human and reproductive rights of women, PAHO was, Morgan argues, 'complicit in perpetuating ignorance, amplifying suffering and ensuring that the worst consequences of the epidemic would be borne by low-income women who lack access to education, medical care and social services for disabled children'.

Mattingly and Keeney Parks (chapter 3) make a remarkable claim about what should be included in a biosocial configuration – or syndemic – that structures experiences of African American families living with a child with autism in Southern California. Few would begin an analysis of such families and their resistance to having their sons labelled autistic by citing statistics of incarceration of Black youth in California. With the stigma attached to the diagnosis? Yes. With the quality of special education classes in public schools in Black communities? Perhaps. But with incarceration? Much more unlikely. Yet this is precisely where the intensive case studies carried out by Mattingly and her colleagues, here represented by two well-educated mothers who strongly resist allowing their children to be diagnosed with autism, took them. This team begins with the data that suggests a puzzling rise to near epidemic proportions of autism in the United States, and hypotheses that range from environmental causes to autism being an 'epidemic of discovery', as the category becomes more well known. But it is the *underdiagnosis* of autism spectrum disorder, ASD, that sets up the paradox that frames this analysis. Mattingly and Keeney Parks respond: 'If health disparities for African Americans are visible as an underdiagnosis when it comes to autism, why are these two mothers so keen to avoid this classification? And why is it worth so much effort? What is so dangerous about it that they devote enormous energy to dodging it? The answer to these questions becomes apparent only when we treat an autism diagnosis in the Black community syndemically, that is, as one element in a configuration in which the epidemic of incarceration plays a pivotal role'. Their intensive case studies took them to the deep awareness of community members of the 'school-to-prison pipeline', particularly for children labelled as troubled and sent to special education classes.

Mattingly and Keeney Parks take up the issue of 'social contagion' for this classic noncommunicable disease. On the one hand, they suggest that in upper middle-class school systems autism is readily diagnosed because the label brings enormous benefits associated with high-quality special education, mandated by school districts, thus encouraging others to seek the diagnosis. But in the schools in the Black community, it is school suspension of Black males at a rate five times greater than for white males, high rates of assignment to juvenile detention facilities, and rates of incarceration five times greater for Black males than those of white males that constitute the contagion leading to this epidemic. None of this is hidden from the eyes of these mothers. And thus it is the experience of being 'haunted by the future' that leads these mothers to so powerfully resist the labelling of their children as autistic.

My reflections here represent only a small part of the fascinating issues raised by the chapters in this volume. Why precisely 'outbreaks' or the rise to epidemic proportions by NCDs occur when they do remains a challenge for research within this paradigm. What exactly constitutes transmissibility or contagion remains to be developed further. The fascinating case of outbreaks of spirit possession, passed from one school child to another as explored by Masquelier and her colleagues (chapter 7) in Niger, reminds us that the label 'mass hysteria' remains a black box for understanding the mysterious power of spirits in many settings in the world, and how the possession of one can lead quickly to the possession of another. The role of individual life histories and personalities linked to susceptibility to particular conditions, such as internet pornography addiction described by anthropologist/psychoanalyst Douglas Hollan (chapter 8), reminds us that why some fall prey to epidemic conditions while others do not is a critical issue for both communicable and noncommunicable conditions. And the relationships between the analyses proposed here and forms of intervention are not fully addressed. Our own work in Aceh (chapter 5) was conducted with the explicit goal of identifying needs for mental health services in a post-conflict setting, which then led us to develop a model of clinical and public mental health interventions. Much of our research, and the analyses that follow, were conducted in the context of providing services to persons self-labelled as suffering from 'trauma'. For the Epicenter paradigm of investigating epidemics, is the development of more effective interventions – clinical, public health, policy – an assumed goal? These and other issues are raised by this fascinating collection of case studies.

Conclusion: Epidemics, Ghosts and Haunting

Eugene Richardson (2020) and Adia Benton (forthcoming) have argued that global public health responses to epidemics, along with epidemiological models, are deeply embedded in colonial histories of 'containment' (Richardson) and 'surveillance, control, and prevention' (Benton). The everyday logics of colonial responses to epidemics, aimed at preventing contagious diseases from the tropics crossing boundaries and making their way into the civilized world, are present in what Richardson calls 'the Coloniality of Global Public Health'. As he writes, 'Since the colonial period in West Africa, the dominant logic for epidemic disease containment (including smallpox, malaria, and influenza) has dictated isolation of sick individuals, with little in the way of patient care' (2020: 33). This logic carried forward into responses to the Ebola epidemic, as Richardson the physician found before meeting Paul Farmer and attaching himself to Partners in Health. But more than this, it carries forward, Richardson (2020: 1) argues, into the very structure of knowledge that assumes global inequality as 'commonsensical' or 'unchangeable facts'. As he argues, 'as an apparatus of *coloniality*, Public Health *manages* (as a profession) and *maintains* (as an academic enterprise) global health inequality' (emphasis in original text). Whether one agrees with this radical critique of global public health or not, it is clear that a history of colonialism haunts the global public health enterprise. This is not unlike the way containment and incarceration haunt responses to African American young men diagnosed with autism in the Los Angeles school system, as described by Mattingly and her colleagues, where mothers are 'haunted by the future'. There is little doubt that epidemics of both infectious diseases and noncommunicable conditions are embedded in 'biosocial configurations'. The question is where our analyses of these conditions are positioned amidst the haunting histories of colonialism, racism, sexism and profound inequities. How do our analyses reproduce biosocial configurations as hegemonic, and how can we better produce analyses grounded in solidarity, in commitment to repair, and in sustained engagement? This is not a critique of the chapters of this volume, authored by many who represent such sustained engagement, but a challenge that grows out of the work represented by this volume, a challenge faced by all of us who work in this field.

Byron J. Good
Professor of Medical Anthropology
Department of Global Health and Social Medicine, Harvard Medical School,
and Department of Anthropology, Harvard University

References

Benton, Adia. Forthcoming. *The Fever Archive*. Minneapolis: University of Minnesota Press.

Desjarlais, Robert, et al. 1995. *World Mental Health: Problems and Priorities in Low-Income Countries*. Oxford: Oxford University Press.

Richardson, Eugene T. 2020. *Epidemic Illusions: On the Coloniality of Global Public Health*. Cambridge, MA: MIT Press.

Rosenberg, Charles E. 1992. *Explaining Epidemics and Other Studies in the History of Medicine*. Cambridge: Cambridge University Press.

Singer, Merill, and Scott Clair. 2003. 'Syndemics and Public Health: Reconceptualizing Disease in Bio-Social Context', *Medical Anthropology Quarterly* 17(4): 423–41.

Index

A
Aarhus Center for Cultural Epidemics, 13, 229, 248, 251, 256
abortion, 12, 17 213–24
Aceh, 15, 124–39, 253, 256
Acholi, 25–28, 30–31, 36–37, 39–40, 144–46, 155–56, 172, 251–53
activists, 71, 124–25, 130, 134–38, 215, 217, 220
   health activists, 124–25, 137–38
   trauma activists, 134–35
ADHD. *See* attention deficit hyperactivity disorder
affect, 4–5, 8, 13, 15, 23, 27–28, 103, 105, 108–9, 113, 151, 172, 175–76, 178, 182, 184–87, 253
affection, 8–9, 14–15, 100, 102–4, 107–10, 114–15, 118–19, 180
   indeterminacy, 14, 102–3, 107, 119, 125
   intersubjectivity, 14, 102–3, 107–8, 119, 174–75
affliction, 15–16, 144–45, 147–49, 153–55, 160–61, 170, 172, 174, 176, 181, 184
African Americans, 14, 68–73, 75–78, 80, 90–91, 254, 256
AIDS, 29, 31, 157, 217. *See also* HIV
alcohol, 13, 23, 30, 34, 41, 52, 109, 148
   abuse, 30
   alcoholism, 5, 25, 107, 146, 251
   consumption, 41

American Convention on Human Rights, 220–21
AMR. *See* antimicrobial resistance
amwuunamwuun, 53, 55–57, 59, 61–62
anaemia, 5
anger, 13, 23–25, 27–30, 32–37, 41, 53, 133, 144, 179
animisme, 180
antibiotics, 228, 231, 253
antimicrobial resistance, 10, 228–29, 231, 253
ASD. *See* autism spectrum disorder
aspirations, 5, 40, 50, 81, 183
asthma, 5, 236
atmosphere, 9, 108–9, 230
attention deficit hyperactivity disorder, 4, 9, 12 82–85, 88
autism, 4, 9, 12, 14, 68–71, 75–78, 82–86, 88, 92–93, 124, 249, 254–55, 257
   autism spectrum disorder, 14, 69–70, 72, 82–83, 254
   as contagion, 70–71

B
bacteria, 1 4, 6, 17, 228–29, 232–33, 241–42, 253
Bateson, Gregory, 8
hooks, bell, 86
belonging, 8, 14, 37, 39, 41, 57, 59–60, 103, 107, 117
biopolitical analyses, 251
biomedicine, 6, 146–47, 149, 155, 159, 168, 181, 223, 229–30

Index

biosocial, 1–2, 4–8, 10, 13–14, 17–18, 62–63, 71, 103, 119, 124, 148, 215, 224, 231, 241, 249–54, 257
  configurations, 4, 215, 224, 250–54, 257
  contagion, 2, 4–5, 7–8, 10, 17, 119
biosociality, 71
Black
  children, 72–75, 84, 91
  communities, 69–70, 91, 254–55
  males, 72–73, 80, 84–85, 92, 255
  students, 73, 75
body, 7–9, 24, 50 63, 86, 104, 107, 110, 113–15, 117–18, 130, 144, 147, 150–52, 156–57 161, 169, 171–73, 176, 183, 185–86, 188, 199, 202–3, 231, 234, 237–38
Bohannon, Paul, 27–29
brokerage, 137–38
  health brokers, 137
  trauma brokers, 138

C

cancer, 3–6, 11
choice, 11, 217
chronic conditions. *See* chronic disease
chronic disease, 3, 76, 244
chronic illness. *See* chronic disease
Chua, Jocelyn, 40, 50
Chuuk, 13, 45, 47–49, 52–58, 60–63
circulating affliction, 16, 170
Clair, Scott, 6, 249
code switching, 78
collective preconscious, 197, 207
colonialism, 28, 31, 41, 45–46, 63, 75, 250, 252–53, 256–57
  coloniality, 252, 256
  post-colonialism, 41, 45–46, 61–62, 251–52
communicable disease, 1, 3–4, 229, 241, 248–49, 256. *See also* infectious disease
communication, 2, 8, 148, 201
Community Mental Health Nursing, 138
co-morbidity, 3, 6, 12

comparison, 44–47, 62, 254
configuration, 1–6, 8–18, 23, 26–29, 33, 35, 37, 39–41, 44–47, 51, 57, 61–63, 68–70, 72, 78, 80, 83–84, 91–92, 100, 103, 107, 110, 113–15, 118–19, 124, 144, 147–49, 153–57, 159–60, 186, 193–95, 200–1, 206–7, 209–10, 213–16, 220, 224, 228–32, 235, 238–39, 241, 243–44, 249–55, 257
  analyses, 10, 148, 160, 195, 228, 249, 254
  theories, 6, 10, 13, 249
conflict, 15–16, 25, 30, 35, 37, 53, 146, 152, 157, 160, 169–71, 178, 204, 256
  armed conflict, 31, 124–29, 130–31, 133–39, 251
  family conflict, 26, 60, 105, 111, 118, 195, 200, 202, 207, 209–10, 238
  gender conflict, 13, 25, 32–34, 41
contagion, 1–2, 4–18, 23, 27, 62–63, 68, 70–72, 76, 81–82, 85–86, 100–3, 105, 107, 108, 118–19, 124–25, 128, 132, 134, 138–39, 147–48, 154, 156, 161, 166–67, 170–78, 182, 184–87, 193–95, 200–1, 206–10, 213–15, 220, 223–24, 230, 232, 241, 249–51, 255–56
  'affective contagion', 166, 182, 184–85
  biosocial contagion, 2, 4–5, 7–8, 10, 17, 119
  contagious disease, 7, 256
  social contagion, 4–5, 7–10, 14, 17, 85, 100–3, 119, 123, 125, 148, 154, 177, 184, 195, 201, 206, 208–10, 223–24, 249–50, 255
  theories, 6, 13, 177, 249
  trauma contagion, 124, 132, 134, 138–39
containment, 252, 256
contamination, 6, 9–10, 13, 15–17, 23, 27–28, 39–41, 78, 123,

260

147–48, 150, 152, 154–57, 161, 169–70, 172, 174, 182, 193–94, 201, 230, 233, 238, 241, 249
context, 5–6, 10, 12–13, 23, 44–47, 51, 56, 59–60, 62–63, 68, 128–29, 136, 139, 148–49, 155, 160, 173, 176, 184, 195, 198, 215, 229, 241–42, 249, 253–254, 256
contraception, 17, 213–17, 219, 222–23
control, 2, 3, 17, 31, 32, 35, 51, 176, 193–94, 198, 213–14, 217, 219–20, 228, 231, 234–35, 241, 242, 244, 252, 256
conversion disorder, 169–71
corona. *See* coronavirus
coronavirus, 2–3, 229, 243–44, 250. *See also* Covid-19
Costa Rica, 220
Covid-19, 1, 3, 243–44, 249–50. *See also* coronavirus

D
DeLanda, Manuel, 230
dengue fever, 5
Denmark, 12, 14, 100, 119, 253
depression, 5–6, 9, 16, 25, 132, 134–36, 146, 149, 192, 201–5, 207, 210, 237, 242–43, 251–52
Derrida, Jacques, 74, 229, 232–34, 253
diabetes, 3, 9, 11, 111, 123
diagnosis, 14, 69–73, 76, 78, 82–85, 92–93, 129, 134, 157–58, 167, 169–70, 231, 236, 254–55
diagnostics, 4, 9–10, 70–71, 75, 83–84, 91, 157, 169, 236, 242
diagnostic systems, 4
Dilley, Roy, 229
discrimination, 17, 219, 224
Dolan, Chris, 30–31, 33, 40
dominatrix, 204–5, 207–9
drawings, 102–6, 108–12, 114–16, 118–19
DRTB. *See* drug-resistant tuberculosis

drug-resistant tuberculosis, 3, 12, 17–18, 228–29, 231–43, 249, 253

E
ecology, 7–8, 12–13, 27, 169
economy, 2, 12, 30, 39, 45, 50–52, 72, 104, 183, 198–200, 209, 220, 235, 242, 252–53
eco-syndemic, 12
education, 3, 17, 49, 69–74, 78–79, 82–87, 92–93, 113, 139, 158, 167, 171, 173, 182–84, 187–88, 198–99, 213–15, 219, 234, 242, 254–55
environment, 2, 5–6, 8–10, 12, 27, 39, 70, 83, 86–87, 92, 104, 108, 124, 148, 171–72, 194–95, 230–31, 241, 254
Epicenter. *See* Aarhus Center for Cultural Epidemics
epidemics, 1–14, 17–18, 25, 27, 29, 44–48, 50–51, 55, 61, 63, 68–73, 92, 99, 101–5, 124–25, 132, 139, 165, 170, 174, 180, 186, 195, 213–20, 223–24, 229–31, 239, 243–44, 248–57
  biosocial, 1, 8, 13–14, 18, 63
  epidemics of attention, 4
  epidemic of incarceration, 14, 70, 72, 92, 255
epigenetics, 5
epistemology, 6–7, 11–12, 14, 51, 57, 62–63, 69, 78, 149, 155, 159–60, 223, 250
everyday life, 58, 145, 159
exorcism, 153, 168–69, 179, 181
experience-near, 6, 13, 15, 23, 51, 103
explanatory model, 6, 149, 230

F
family, 8, 12, 14–16, 24, 26–28, 30–31, 33–39, 41, 48, 53–54, 58, 60–61, 75, 78, 87, 93, 100, 103–6, 108–19, 144–45, 147–53, 155, 160, 200, 204,

209, 231, 234, 237–39, 241, 253. *See also* kinship
fantasy, 16–17, 127, 194–200, 202–10
fear, 3, 8, 11–12, 15, 29, 36, 52, 83, 92, 133, 136, 169, 179, 183–84, 195, 198, 203, 217, 223–24
filiation of children, 35, 41
Finnström, Sverker, 39–40
Foster, Paula Hirsch, 27–28, 30–32, 39
Foucault, 11, 215, 251
Free Aceh Movement, 126–27, 137. *See also* Aceh
Freud, Sigmund, 195–98, 207, 210

G
GAM. *See* Free Aceh Movement
gender, 4, 13, 23–26, 28, 33, 35, 37–41, 56, 78, 107, 110, 175, 183–84, 214–15, 219–20, 222, 224, 242
  gender pattern, 23, 28
génies tchatcheurs, 169, 171, 182. *See also* iskoki, jinn
ghosts, 25, 27, 75, 156, 248, 256
  ghosts of colonial and racialized pasts, 250
Girling, Frank, 31
global gag rule, 221–22
global health, 12, 124, 221–22, 251, 256
Grøn, Lone, 14–15, 124, 253

H
haunting, 5, 8, 14–16, 75, 92, 103, 115, 118–19, 147, 156, 158, 185–88, 193–94, 200, 206–7, 209, 250, 256–57
  'haunted by the future', 14, 68, 73, 255, 257
  haunted buildings, 168–69, 171–72, 178, 182, 185–86
  hauntological analyses, 251
  hauntology, 14, 74–75
health agencies, 17, 223
health systems, 4, 136, 158, 238
heart disease, 5

Helsinki Memorandum of Understanding, 126
heritage, 25, 33 104, 186, 188, 203
high blood pressure, 9
hijab, 176, 185, 188
HIV, 4, 6, 31, 157, 217, 222. *See also* AIDS
Holý, Ladislav, 229
homeplace, 70, 86–88, 90–92
  limits of homeplace, 90
human rights, 129, 183, 214, 216, 219–24
humanitarian aid, 129–30
hygge, 103, 106, 108, 110–11, 119, 253
hypertension. *See* high blood pressure

I
iconoclasm, 168, 181
imitation, 4, 7–8, 16, 81, 165, 170, 177–78, 187
immodesty, 169, 176, 185
immunity, 9, 150, 186–87
incarceration, 14, 69–70, 72–73, 92, 254–56
India, 3, 12, 17, 50, 232, 234–36, 241, 244, 254
individuality, 173, 187
Indonesia, 12, 15, 125–27, 129, 133–34, 136–39
inequality, 1, 6, 46, 56, 103, 118, 181, 183, 220, 244, 256–57
infection, 1, 4, 6, 10, 12, 17, 68, 77, 213, 218, 223, 236, 249, 254
infectious disease, 1, 3–4, 6, 7, 12, 231, 249, 257. *See also* communicable disease
International Organization for Migration, 125, 127–28, 131, 134–35, 137
internet porn, 16, 193–95, 197, 199–201, 206–7, 249, 255
IOM. *See* International Organization for Migration
iskoki, 178–79. *See also génies tchatcheurs*, jinn)
Islam, 168, 179–81, 183
Izala, 168–69, 181

malamai, 180
Qur'an as protection, 168–69
Qur'anic medicine, 168, 171
Issacs, Susan, 196

J
jinn, 167–68, 178–79, 186. *See also génies tchatcheurs, iskoki*)

K
kinship, 8, 104–5, 110, 118. *See also* family
kinship connection, 8, 118
Kizza, Dorothy, 31, 33, 40
Klein, Melanie, 196

L
Latin America, 12, 17, 213, 215–17, 223–24
life conditions, 11–12, 31, 68, 72
lifestyle, 11, 15, 101, 103, 118–19, 159, 194
lifestyle diseases, 11, 100
Livingston, Julie, 30, 40
Lord's Resistance Army, 25, 32, 144–45, 157, 251
love, 4, 8, 14, 38, 58–59, 61, 75, 103–4, 107, 110, 119, 169–70, 202, 234
LRA. *See* Lord's Resistance Army
lung cancer, 5, 11

M
malaria, 5, 256
marriage, 23–24, 31–33, 35–38, 91, 115, 168, 181, 183, 185, 204, 234, 238, 253
masculinity, 13, 23, 29–32
mass hysteria, 167, 169, 174, 184, 187, 255. *See also* mass possession, spiritual attacks
mass incarceration, 68, 72, 92
material conditions, 10
materiality, 9, 12, 155–56
Meinert, Lotte, 15, 63, 81, 103, 124, 145, 172, 195, 201, 251
mental health, 14, 44, 69, 71, 83, 125–27, 129, 131–32, 134–39, 146, 158, 202, 210, 251–52, 256
mental health problems, 134, 139, 158, 249, 251, 253
mental health services, 125, 127, 134, 139, 256
metaphor, 3–4, 13–14, 48, 51, 62, 74, 81, 186, 248–49
microbes. *See* bacteria
microcephaly, 213, 215–18, 223, 254
micro-organisms, 6–7, 249
mind, 7–8, 52, 54, 77, 158, 171–72, 200, 242
mindful body, 7, 9
minority communities, 14
mood, 8, 108, 147, 187, 240
moral breakdown, 59–60, 62
Morrison, Toni, 75
mutuality, 14, 18, 103, 111, 187, 202, 241, 243

N
NCD. *See* noncommunicable diseases
network, 12, 48, 59–62, 102, 104–6, 109, 111–12, 115–16, 137, 166, 175
NGO. *See* nongovernmental organization
Niehaus, Isak, 29
noncommunicable disease, 1, 3, 9, 68, 81, 124, 186, 247–49, 255
nongovernmental organization, 16, 125, 128, 137, 145–46, 157–60, 183, 222
nutrition, 4, 8

O
obesity, 3–5, 11–12, 14–15, 100–8, 110–13, 115–16, 118–19, 248–49, 253
as epidemic, 3–5, 11, 14–15, 100, 102–5, 124, 248
Obeyesekere, Gananath, 196, 208
Oceania, 12–14, 44–45, 47–48, 50–51, 55–57, 60, 62, 252
ordinary affects, 166, 185, 187

Index

P

PAHO. *See* Pan American Health Organization
Pan American Health Organization, 213–15, 217–24, 254
pandemic, 1–3, 229, 244, 249–51
permeability, 9, 175–76, 187
pharmakon, 232–36, 241–43
phenomenology, 14, 57, 63, 74, 77–78, 102, 119, 124, 129–30, 134, 148–49, 201
PNA. *See* psychosocial needs assessment
poisonous knowledge, 133
policy, 5, 11, 61, 72, 136–37, 148, 215, 218–19, 221–22, 224, 241–44, 249–50, 253–54, 256
political economy, 13, 23, 68
porn addiction, 12, 193, 255
Porter, Holly, 28
possession, 4–5, 16, 146, 166–80, 182, 185–87, 255
  ceremonies, 168
  episodes, 167, 169
  mass possession, 16, 167, 170–71, 173, 178, 180, 182, 185–87 (*see also* spiritual attacks, mass hysteria)
  as resistance, 168, 170, 173, 187
  of schoolgirls, 16, 165, 167–71, 73, 180, 186–87
post-conflict, 15, 124–25, 127–29, 131, 136–37, 139, 146, 160, 256
post-traumatic stress disorder, 4, 6, 9–10, 130, 132, 134–36, 146–47, 154, 157–59
post-tsunami, 15, 124–25, 127, 139
pregnancy, 17, 107, 213–23
  pregnancy termination (*see* abortion)
privilege, 28, 63, 177, 199–200, 207, 209
protection, 9, 14, 24, 26, 30, 34, 69–70, 73, 77, 84–85, 91–92, 118, 130, 148, 168, 176, 180–81, 183, 185–86, 216, 221, 223–24

psychoanalysis, 193–94, 196, 210, 255
psychosocial needs assessment, 125, 128, 131–34, 137
PTSD. *See* post-traumatic stress disorder
puskesmas, 127, 134, 136–37, 139

R

reconfiguration. *See* configuration
regimen, 17, 232–37, 239–42, 244
relationality, 174, 184
repetition, 7, 49, 177, 194, 198, 207
reproductive governance, 17, 213, 215, 224
reproductive health, 214–24
resistance, 3, 9–10, 12, 16–18, 25, 36, 73, 86, 90, 144–45, 150, 168, 170, 173, 187, 228–38, 240–43, 249, 251, 253–55
resonance, 4, 8, 47, 57, 58, 77, 101, 147–48, 165, 172–74, 176, 178, 185–87, 197, 204, 207
Rosenberg, Charles, 6, 10, 27–29, 92, 148, 230–31, 249

S

schoolgirls, 16, 166–71, 173, 175, 178–80, 183–87
Seeberg, Jens, 17, 63, 81, 103, 124, 195, 227, 229, 253
self, 8–9, 11, 52, 57, 62, 78, 110, 133, 150, 157, 177–78, 187, 252
self-harm, 5, 26, 50–53, 56–57, 60–61, 252
sexuality, 194, 199, 205–6, 210, 215
sexually transmitted infections, 213
Singer, Merrill, 6, 12, 68, 74, 249
social constellations, 250
social harmony, 28, 35
social order, 10, 224
socioeconomic, 3, 6–7, 11–12, 209, 241
Socrates, 232
space-of-relating, 57
spirit possession, 4–5, 16, 146, 166, 168, 170–71, 175, 186–87, 255

spiritual attacks, 166–67, 169–70, 172, 174–76, 178–79, 182, 185–87, 249. *See also* mass possession, mass hysteria
Stewart, Kathleen, 185, 187
stigma, 8, 15, 17, 70–71, 77, 84–85, 87, 93, 102, 125, 130, 136, 139, 216, 242, 254
suicide, 4–5, 12–14, 23–41, 44–63, 107, 146, 237–38, 243, 247, 249, 251–53
　endemic suicide, 48, 51
　epidemic readings of, 13, 47, 50, 55, 61
　epidemic suicide, 43, 47, 62, 252
　as social practice, 45, 57
　suicide attempts, 26, 36, 51, 52, 252
surveillance, 134, 215, 256
syndemics, 3, 6–7, 10, 12, 14, 18, 68–70, 72, 74–75, 81–82, 92–93, 243, 249, 254–255

T

Tarde, Gabriel, 7–8, 16, 170, 177–78, 182, 184, 187
TB. *See* tuberculosis
torture, 126, 128–29, 131–32, 146, 156
toxicity, 169, 182, 233–36, 238, 240–43
trauma, 4, 12, 15–16, 25, 75, 103, 124–25, 127–39, 145–48, 155, 157–61, 169, 171, 195, 200, 209–10, 249, 251, 253, 256
　collective trauma, 138
　secondary trauma, 133
treatment, 3, 11, 16, 26, 31, 71, 127, 134–36, 139, 146–47, 149, 151–53, 155, 157–60, 167, 169, 205, 215, 222, 224, 231, 233–45, 251–52

tsunami, 15, 124–27, 136, 138–39
　Indian Ocean Tsunami, 125–126
tuberculosis, 3, 12, 17, 228–29, 231–33, 241, 249, 253

U

Uganda, 9, 12–13, 15, 23, 25, 28, 30–31, 40–41, 144–47, 153, 155–58, 160, 172, 251, 253

V

violence, 8, 15–16, 24–26, 29, 36, 74–75, 80, 124–32, 134, 136–38, 143, 145–51, 153–55, 158–61, 167, 172, 182, 220, 222, 237, 251, 253
　political violence, 124, 129, 138
　remainders of violence, 125, 131, 136, 138
virus, 1–5, 10, 12, 17, 213–16, 218–19, 221–24, 229, 232–33, 243–44, 249–50, 254
vulnerability, 3, 18, 40, 50, 130, 150, 175–76, 179, 194, 198, 207, 223, 243

W

Waldenfels, Bernhard, 102
war, 13, 15, 23, 25, 30–32, 35, 39–41, 55, 72, 125, 128–32, 144–45, 148, 152–53, 157, 160, 251, 253
Weber, Max, 11
WHO. *See* World Health Organization
World Health Organization, 28, 213, 216, 219, 221–22 231, 234, 236, 244

Z

Zika virus, 5, 12, 17, 213–24, 249, 254

www.ingramcontent.com/pod-product-compliance
Lightning Source LLC
Chambersburg PA
CBHW051532020426
42333CB00016B/1897